How to Quit Drugs for Good

A Complete Self-Help Guide

Jerry Dorsman

THREE RIVERS PRESS
NEW YORK

Copyright © 1998 by Jerry Dorsman

Published by Three Rivers Press, New York, New York. Member of the Crown Publishing Group, a division of Random House, Inc. www.crownpublishing.com

THREE RIVERS PRESS and the Tugboat design are registered trademarks of Random House, Inc.

Originally published by Prima Publishing, Roseville, California, in 1998.

Drug addiction is a serious matter. Readers should seek medical and/or psychological counseling if they suffer from drug addiction. This book is not intended to be a substitute for such counseling.

"Chapter 14: Zig Ziglar's Seven Steps to Achieving Goals" from *Goals*, copyright © 1986, Zig Ziglar. By permission Nightingale-Conant Corporation.

Printed in the United States of America

Library of Congress Cataloging-in-Publication Data

Dorsman, Jerry.
    How to quit drugs for good : a complete self-help guide / Jerry Dorsman.
        p.   cm.
    Includes bibliographical references and index.
        1. Drug abuse—United States—Prevention.   2. Drug abuse—Treatment—United States.   3. Narcotic addicts—Rehabilitation—United States.   4. Self-help techniques—United States.   I. Title.
HV5825.D675 1998
613.8'3—dc21   98-40638
                                                                       CIP

ISBN 0-7615-1517-8

10 9

First Edition

*To each and every person
who chooses to quit using drugs . . .
This book is dedicated to your success.*

Contents

Acknowledgements

My Special Thanks . . .

To Andrew Vallas, assistant project editor at Prima Publishing, for managing the editorial process with verve and efficiency, and to Bruce Owens, copy editor, for upgrading the quality of the final text.

To Sean Goodwin for his editorial advice on key portions of the text.

To my wife, Kathy Cunningham, for her editorial advice on the text and for her emotional support throughout the project.

To Ben Dominitz, president at Prima Publishing, for recommending that I do this book and for supporting the project financially.

To Richard H. Bayer, Ph.D., CEO, at Upper Bay Counseling and Support Services, Inc., for his ongoing friendship and for allowing me the freedom to change my hours at work.

To Robert Wilson, Psy.D., my clinical supervisor at UBCSS, for helping me to improve my psychotherapy skills with clients.

And to my mom, Ruth Mae Dorsman, for the loving, caring environment she created for me in my youth. The memory of this through the years has lifted me, more than once, from the depths of despair. I thank her too for her friendship in recent years and for being a loving grandmother to my children.

Preface

When the publisher of my first two books urged me to write a book on quitting drugs, I didn't jump at the idea. "After all," I told him, "the methods which help people quit drugs are just about the same as those which help people quit drinking. And I've already described all of those methods in my first book, *How to Quit Drinking Without AA.*"

"I know," he said, "but people who have a problem with drugs would not pick up a book that tells them how to quit drinking." He had a point.

I thought about it. In addition, I began to do some research. I learned that nearly 75 million Americans have used an illicit drug at least once in their lifetimes. Of this group, about 13 million, or 6% of the total U.S. population, are current users. Moreover, drug use among teenagers has grown to epidemic proportions, and this trend continues.

So, within a couple of months, I changed my mind. I decided to write this book. Not only were the numbers greater than what I had thought; my publisher was also right. People with drug addictions could use a book that was written specifically to help them break these addictions.

Now, I offer this book to you as a potential resource. On these pages, you'll find a complete step-by-step program that will help you become drug free—and stay that way. If you have a problem with drugs, this book can help you quit.

So here's a chance to renew yourself. By reading this guidebook and following its methods, you can make a major change—a change that will last the rest of your life. When you choose to become drug free by using these methods, you'll boost your energy, find greater happiness, and add many wholesome years to your life.

The time to start is now.

Introduction

How This Book Can Help

Nearly every day, we hear something more about society's "War on Drugs." Newspapers and magazines routinely barrage us with new details of America's "drug epidemic." Government officials and local school board administrators call for more drug prevention programs in the schools.

What is happening? Can our drug problem be so big that we need an all-out war to fight it?

There are different points of view concerning drugs. Many people ask, "What's the matter with catching a little buzz now and then?" This is a common question. You'll hear it especially among those who've just started into treatment for a drug problem.

Yet answering this question can be difficult. To be realistic, we must answer, "Maybe nothing." Maybe there's nothing wrong with catching a little buzz now and then. But we need to be specific. Maybe nothing's wrong if it's really only a little buzz, if it's really only now and then, and if it's not causing some kind of problem in our lives. A morning cup of coffee once a week would qualify.

Of course, it's not easy to content ourselves with little buzzes. Many of us go for bigger and bigger buzzes, perhaps even a veritable din of buzzes. Some of us will settle for nothing less than having a blast. And it's not easy to limit ourselves. If something gives us a rush, some overwhelming sense of pleasure however brief, we want to do it again. And again. We don't care to wait. And once we start going for it, going for the buzzes and pleasures in a big way, these substances—no matter how innocent they might seem—begin to cause problems in our lives.

Recent statistics from the Substance Abuse and Mental Health Services Administration (SAMHSA) of the U.S. Department of Health and Human Services show that nearly five million people have, at least some time in their lives, entered treatment for a drug problem. This is just the number who entered treatment.

How many more have a problem with drugs who didn't enter treatment? SAMHSA's *National Household Survey on Drug Abuse* (1996) showed that 23 million Americans had used some variety of illicit drug during the past year. What was counted as an illicit drug? Marijuana, cocaine, heroin, hallucinogens, phencyclidines (PCP), methamphetamine, inhalants, and the nonmedical use of psychotherapeutics (e.g., stimulants, sedatives, tranquilizers, and analgesics). Among this 23 million, 3.8 million were teenagers, aged 12 to 17.

The same survey revealed that more than 13 million people used an illicit drug during the past month, a figure that included more than two million teenagers. Any or all of these 13 million "current users" could have some kind of problem with drugs.

THINGS HAVEN'T ALWAYS BEEN THIS WAY

Sixty-five years ago, hardly anyone used illicit drugs. A few people used reefer. A few people were hooked on morphine. Most of them were started on it for a medical reason—to kill pain. A few people were hooked on barbiturates. Again, most had been started on it medically—to help with sleep. Only one person had tripped on LSD, Dr. Albert Hoffmann, who ingested it inadvertently in 1938 after he had synthesized it at Sandoz Laboratories in Switzerland. Hardly anyone was addicted to cocaine. In fact, an initial wave of cocaine use had already come and gone. From the late 1800s to the early 1900s, cocaine had appeared as a key ingredient in numerous "medical" tonics (including Coca-Cola from 1886 to 1903), and a small but significant percentage of people got hooked on these. The smokable forms of cocaine, known as freebase and crack, had not yet been invented. Hardly anyone had touched heroin. A small percentage of people were hooked on amphetamines, primarily because of a popular bronchial dilator known as the "Benzedrine inhaler," developed by Smith, Kline, and French and available in the 1930s and 1940s. It became known on the street as the "B-Bomb." Tranquilizers had not been developed yet, nor had PCP. If anyone got high from inhaling solvents (e.g., glue or gasoline), it was almost always a mistake, usually from working too long around these substances in an enclosed area.

Sixty-five years ago, the main drugs of choice were the legal ones—alcohol, tobacco, and caffeine. They were all used by significant percentages of people. But whatever drug people chose to use, the people doing the choosing were almost invariably adults, over the age of 18.

In the 1950s, drug use began to increase. Marijuana led the way. It started among young adults, people mainly in their twenties, often in college or just graduated from college. A key segment of this group who popularized the use of marijuana called themselves "beatniks." During the beatnik era, smoking opium and using one of its derivatives, heroin, became popular, but only on a small scale and once again only among adults.

During the 1960s, things changed dramatically. In this decade, we witnessed significant increases in the use of nearly all classes of illicit drugs. This was the era of the "hippies." It too began among young adults—people who had already graduated high school. By the late 1960s, a whole generation—nearly everyone aged 18 to 25—had tried, or were currently using, some kind of mind-altering drug. The leading edge of the baby-boom generation, these folks could be found almost everywhere, from the back streets of big cities to college campuses.

In the 1970s, the hippies' quest for peace, love, and flower power continued. Not only did more and more young adults begin using drugs, but more and more older children began using them. It was during this era that we witnessed a steady lowering of the "age of entry," and by the late 1970s drug use had become common among high schoolers.

In the 1980s, the age of entry into the drug scene dropped even further. During this decade, drug use became even more common among high schoolers but also had started a trend among middle schoolers. Today, significant percentages of middle schoolers have tried, or have begun using, at least one illicit drug.

Also, there's another key trend. From the 1970s to the present, people in all age-groups have begun using a greater variety of drugs. In terms of the numbers of people who have used one or more illicit drugs, marijuana leads the way, followed by cocaine, hallucinogens, inhalants, analgesics, amphetamines and other stimulants, tranquilizers, PCP, sedatives, and heroin. Based on SAMHSA's 1996 survey on drug abuse, the following percentages of Americans have used the following drugs at some time during their lives: 34.8% (marijuana), 10.3% (cocaine), 9.7% (hallucinogens), 5.6% (inhalants), 5.5% (analgesics, i.e., painkillers), 4.7% (amphetamines or other stimulants), 3.6% (tranquilizers), 3.2% (PCP), 2.3% (sedatives), and 1.1% (heroin). This comprises the list of drugs that you'll find specifically detailed in this book. However, I've also included some information on alcohol, nicotine, caffeine, and over-the-counter medications, especially concerning their role in the use of, and recovery from, drugs.

Clearly, our society has changed in many ways. During the past 50 years, an ever greater number of people have begun using an ever greater variety of drugs. This has become most obvious among people in the younger generations. Indeed, their whole world has changed. In his book *Familyhood*, Dr. Lee Salk reported the top seven school problems of the 1940s: talking in class, chewing gum, making noise, running in the halls, cutting into line, dress-code violations, and littering. He then compared these to the top seven school problems of the 1990s: drug abuse, alcohol abuse, pregnancy, suicide, rape, robbery, and assault. Of course, a person's involvement in the first two problems of the 1990s (drug and alcohol abuse) often leads to the other problems (pregnancy, suicide, rape, robbery, and assault). What might help in our schools? What might help in our society? Would it help if more people decided to quit using drugs?

Would it help you in any way if you could quit using drugs?

APPROACHES TO QUITTING

If you've ever tried quitting drugs, you know it can be difficult. In fact, without the right approach, it can be nearly impossible. What's the right approach? The right approach is whatever's "right for you."

Each person needs to find his or her own way. The best approach for you will be the one that feels comfortable to you and that offers techniques suited to your individual needs. But it's up to you to learn what will work for you. You must decide.

Many programs have been proven to work. Yet treatment professionals still recommend one specific program, Narcotics Anonymous (NA), more than any other. Unfortunately, many drug users who want to quit don't want to join NA. They don't like NA's approach for one reason or another. You might feel this way, too. Here are the two main reasons people give for disliking NA:

1. NA bases its program on a specific religious and moral philosophy. If the philosophy doesn't match your own, you're more likely to fail, no matter how hard you try. Part of this approach requires a moralistic attitude that many people aren't willing to adopt.

2. NA offers group therapy with a social support network. This can be very successful for those who feel comfortable in groups. However, many drug-dependent individuals feel extremely anxious in a group. These people can't function in a group unless they're high.

There's one other problem with NA. Along with its parent organization, Alcoholics Anonymous (AA), it has been stubbornly resistant to change. The Twelve Step program has remained basically the same since its inception in 1935. Even when new discoveries show how recovering individuals can improve their health, AA and NA haven't incorporated these techniques into their programs. In fact, AA and NA neglect to offer any information on how to treat the physical damage caused by addiction.

But repairing the body must be an essential goal of recovery. This becomes clear when you consider that drug addiction is a biological disorder causing damage to every one of the body's cells. The ongoing cellular damage leads to numerous diseases with serious physical and mental side effects. When you quit drugs, you can improve dramatically by using healing techniques that repair this damage.

Other important treatment goals include the fulfillment of your social, emotional, and spiritual needs. To meet these other needs, it helps if you have a variety of options. That way, you can choose the options best suited to your nature.

A NEW SELF-HELP APPROACH

At present, many programs offer alternative approaches to breaking a drug addiction. Many of these new alternatives, including the self-help approach in this book, allow you to choose your own specific techniques. Within a given framework, you discover what works for you and then begin to use it. In this way, you plan an approach uniquely suited to your needs.

The self-help approach in this book is based on one simple premise: *You can take responsibility for your own health.* By doing so, not only will you want to stop taking drugs but you also will learn how. Once you know the specific problems you need to overcome and the best methods for achieving your goals, you can do this with relative ease. With this book you will examine your individual need for drugs, decide when to quit, develop your own treatment plan, choose the techniques that will work for you, and create your own success.

It's up to you. This self-help approach offers you everything you need—the latest facts, the best new treatment methods, and an organized plan to guide you. Now, more than ever before, you can choose to help yourself.

PART ONE

WHAT DO DRUGS MEAN TO YOU?

CHAPTER 1

Drugs of Abuse

*Everything is a dangerous drug except reality,
which is unendurable.*
> —Cyril Connolly

*The universal human need for liberation
from . . . mundane existence is satisfied by
experiencing altered states of consciousness.
. . . Some follow the paths of prayer or meditation in their quest for spiritual insight, while
others are transported to the higher planes by
way of ecstasies induced by art, music, sexual
passion or intoxicating substances.*
> —Richard Rudgley

In our society we have available to us a wide array of substances. From the corner drugstore to the dealer in the streets, we can find almost anything. But what makes some substances more attractive than others? Why do some become "drugs of abuse?"

Every substance with psychoactive traits has the potential to become a drug of abuse. A psychoactive substance, when we take it, changes our consciousness. That is, it changes the way things appear to us or the way we feel.

Of course, this result can hold a powerful attraction for us. How completely compelling! If the world seems dull, we merely need to take some magic potion to make things come alive again. Simple. Easy.

Perhaps too easy.

Perhaps too compelling. We humans can become addicted to substances such as these. We can find ourselves loving the magic so much that we keep coming back for more.

Which many of us do. In our lifetimes nearly every one of us will try at least one psychoactive substance. Most of us will stick to drugs that are legal. For example, the mild stimulant caffeine, found in coffee, tea, chocolate, and soft drinks, has become one of the most widely used psychoactive substances in the world.

But in our lifetimes, about 35% of us in the United States will try at least one illicit drug—marijuana, cocaine, heroin, PCP, methamphetamine, an inhalant, a hallucinogen, or the nonmedical use of a psychotherapeutic (e.g., stimulant, sedative, tranquilizer, or analgesic). About 11% of us report that we have used at least one of these illicit drugs during the past year, and 6.1%, or more than 13 million, are "current users."

MARIJUANA

Marijuana comes from the hemp plant, *Cannabis sativa*. This plant contains hundreds of chemicals, including more than 60 cannabinoids. The most potent of the cannabinoids is delta-9-tetrahydrocannabinol, or THC.

Except for the cannabinoids, marijuana smoke and tobacco smoke are remarkably similar. Both contain the toxic compounds tar, carbon monoxide, and cyanide in comparable levels. Both also contain benzopyrine, a known cancer-causing chemical. This chemical appears in greater concentrations in marijuana smoke than in tobacco smoke, although marijuana smoke contains none of the nitrosamines found in tobacco.

Options

Marijuana. This product is made of the dried clippings from the hemp plant that may include any combination of leaves, stems, seeds, and buds. It can vary greatly in potency, depending on the type of plant, the climate in which it was grown, and the specific mix of clippings in a given batch. The typical THC concentrations in marijuana are 2% to 5%. This runs somewhat higher than the THC content in the marijuana of the 1960s, which averaged between 0.5% and 3%. More potent forms, such as sinsemilla, can contain 7% THC. Marijuana is also known as (AKA): Cannibis, Pot, Grass, Reefer, Ace, Sinse, Ganja, Weed, Giggle Weed, Tea, Bhang, Doobie, M.J., Mary Jane, Columbian, Acapulco Gold, Mexican, Maui Wowie, Panama Red, Thai Sticks, Indian.

Hashish. People make hashish by separating the resin of a cannabis plant from the plant material. This product averages 5% to 12% THC concentration, and some varieties run as high as 20%. AKA: Hash, Tar.

Hash oil. This oil is produced by extracting the cannabinoids from the pot plant through the use of a solvent such as alcohol. The thick, waxy liquid—which varies in color depending on the solvent used—contains anywhere from 15% to 70% THC. AKA: Honey Oil, Weed Oil.

Synthetic THC. Scientists have developed dronabinol, a product containing synthetic THC, for use with cancer patients in controlling nausea or vomiting caused by chemotherapy agents and to stimulate the appetites of AIDS patients. Trade name: Marinol.

Combinations. Some users will smoke marijuana in combinations with hash or hash oil, with tobacco, or with numerous other drugs. Other drugs (along with street names for the combination) include: phencyclidine (Angel Dust, Angel Poke, Supergrass, Killer Weed), opium (O.J.), heroin (Atom Bomb, A-Bomb), and cocaine or crack (Juice Joint, Lace, Fry Daddy, Cocoa Puff).

How It's Used

Most people get their THC buzz by smoking, that is, by setting flame to their marijuana, hash, or hash oil and inhaling. However, some people will take time to cook one of these three substances into brownies, cakes, or pudding and then eat the results. The user who smokes will experience a high within two to 10 minutes, while the high from eating may take as long as 90 minutes. Synthetic THC (dronabinol) comes in tablets.

Popularity

Somewhere between 30% and 34% of Americans have tried marijuana. About 8.6% have used it within the past year, and 4.7% have used it within the past month. That's the equivalent of about 10.1 million people using pot within the past month. Of these current users, 1.6 million were aged 12 to 17, and 3.7 million were aged 18 to 25.

The Joy of It

There are probably as many different experiences on pot as there are people who have used it, but the high has two distinguishing features: intellectual and emotional. Most people experience one or the other type of high, and some people experience a little of both.

The intellectual type of high can be described as a heightening of awareness. The perceptions from all five senses become more vivid. Everything we see, hear, smell, taste, and touch takes on a greater intensity or somehow seems more meaningful. We become certain that our thoughts are more profound. Our mind appears to make more connections than usual, some of which seem downright funny. We often feel as though we're gaining a greater insight into reality.

The emotional high affects our feelings. Everything we feel becomes exaggerated or all-encompassing. The world becomes a ball of fluff. Pleasures become ecstasies, joys become wonders, smiles become laughs. We like being in the company of others. Talking with others becomes interesting, even mesmerizing. Our moods deserve exploring. People who experience the emotional high enjoy doing things, much more so than those who experience the intellectual high. Perhaps that's because physical activity generates more emotion.

However, the more potent the weed, the more likely that the user will experience some mind-warping effects, such as delusions, hallucinations, or cartoonlike visions. These imaginary sequences come more easily with the eyes closed but, at higher concentrations of THC, can occur with the eyes open. Sometimes, when the images soar, the body feels as if it weighs a ton. At these times, the body can demonstrate a perfect reluctance to make any movement whatsoever. Perhaps this is the original meaning of the term "stoned."

The Problems It Causes

Panic. Many users experience panic attacks. These usually occur in public places where we can be seen by others. Often the panic has a hint of paranoia. For example, users might fear that other people are out to get them, that somehow their behavior will betray to others that they're high, or that the police are coming to bust them for possession. After a moderate period of heavy use (about a year or so) or a longer period of moderate use, the panic response can generalize. In other words, it begins to happen even when the user is not high, and this can continue for years after the user has gotten completely straight.

Anxiety. Many users also experience anxiety. This is similar to the panic attacks, except that it has no object. We can feel jittery, nervous, and tense, and we're not sure why. It appears as a gnawing feeling in the pit of the stomach or a shaky uncertainty within the brain. This anxiety generalizes as well and can continue for years after a user gets straight.

Interestingly, people who get the intellectual kick usually feel more anxious when they use, whereas those who experience the emotional high usually feel less anxious when using.

Learning and memory impairment. Animal studies show that THC causes significant deficits in the brain's ability to store new memories so that learning becomes impaired. This probably happens in humans as well, especially heavy users. Because you wouldn't be able to remember details very well, trying to study while high on pot wouldn't be recommended.

Disruption of logical thought. Trying to do math while high on pot also wouldn't be recommended. Many studies show that pot disrupts our ability to think logically, in other words, to perceive what follows what in sequential events or number patterns. Events run together, and causes and effects become blurred. This problem also generalizes. In the long term, moderate to heavy users lose some of their capability for logic, even when not toking up. This problem can last for years after getting straight, although it typically shows considerable improvement after the first few months.

Psychosis. A small but significant percentage of chronic heavy users will become psychotic. For them, logical thought almost completely disappears. Delusions and hallucinations replace reality. The most typical psychosis for this group is paranoid schizophrenia. In other words, they have persistent notions that people are out to do them some kind of harm but they commonly get all mixed up as to who exactly is out to get them, for what reason, and what it is these people will do.

At the local mental health clinic, I counsel many clients who have been "dual-diagnosed" (i.e., with both a psychosis and an addiction). About 15% of the chronic clients—those who remain mentally ill even after breaking their drug and alcohol addictions—remember their pot use as playing a key role in the onset of the mental illness. They believe that pot use triggered their original break from reality. A few of the acute clients—those in short-term care—have been dual-diagnosed with a psychosis and just one addiction: cannabis dependence. Once these clients quit using pot, their delusions and mental confusions begin to disappear. Often within a month their logical thought improves noticeably, and within a year their overall functioning approaches "normal."

Reduced motivation. Some studies link pot smoking to reduced motivation, or amotivational syndrome.

Users experiencing amotivation will procrastinate, forget, or simply choose not to do certain things. They begin to shirk some of life's key responsibilities. They might do poorly in school or find it difficult to hold a job.

Lung problems. Pot smoking definitely damages the lungs. The lungs of long-term heavy users show decreased airflow compared to the lungs of nonusers. In addition, long-term heavy pot smoking leads to chronic bronchitis and most likely causes lung cancer.

Harm from accidents. Marijuana impairs the user's driving ability and affects actual performance behind the wheel. Each year, thousands of accidents are reported in which the driver at fault was high on marijuana. In some of these accidents, people were killed.

Withdrawal

When coming off pot, you can expect to become irritable, restless, or tense, and when feeling this way you'll crave marijuana. This anxiety response will be mild, moderate, or heavy, depending on whether your habit was mild, moderate, or heavy. It will continue at least for weeks, usually for a few months, or perhaps even longer than a year. As part of the anxiety response, you might also experience insomnia, vivid dreams, or both.

In early recovery, you might experience sweating, mild nausea, or lack of appetite. This can last a few days or as long as a week.

THC remains in the fatty deposits in the body. Because of this, THC and its metabolites can be detected in the body as long as 3 weeks after smoking just one joint and can remain in the body for months after a period of heavy use.

COCAINE

Cocaine comes from the coca plant, *Erythroxylon coca*. Its green leaves contain the nutrients thiamine, riboflavin, and vitamin C and the psychoactive alkaloid cocaine.

For centuries, the indigenous people of the Andes Mountains have eaten coca leaves. They mix the leaves with an alkali (lime) that helps release the cocaine from the roughage. About 90% of the Indians indulge—some of them all day long—but the total amount of stimulant they ingest compares to the amount of stimulant Americans get from drinking coffee. The Indian who chews two ounces of leaves gets about 0.7 grains of cocaine per day. A typical cocaine abuser might take six to eight grains per day, or about 10 times what the Indian ingests.

Options

Cocaine. People make cocaine (known technically as cocaine hydrochloride) through a lengthy process using various chemicals and solvents. Starting with coca leaves and sulfuric acid, producers draw off the liquid and then add more acid, along with lime, water, gasoline, potassium permanganate, and ammonia. This creates a paste that is further refined by using kerosene, methyl alcohol, and more sulfuric acid. The result is the white crystalline powder that has a bitter, numbing effect when tasted. AKA: Coke, Snow, Snow White, Charlie, Toot, Nose Candy, C, C-Dust, Girl, Lady, Lady-Caine.

Crack. Crack is a form of "freebase" but is safer to produce than the original freebase, which required the chemical ether. Crack is made by boiling powdered cocaine with sodium bicarbonate. This "frees" the cocaine "base" from the cocaine hydrochloride. The base separates from solution as chunks of crack. AKA: Rock, Hard Rock, Pebbles, Stones, Gravel, Baby T, Cookies, Fries, Fifty-One, One-Fifty-One, Pony, White Ghost, Sleet.

Combinations. Some users will inject a combination of cocaine and heroin (AKA: Speedball, Dynamite, Murder One, Whizz-Bang). Some users will smoke crack with other smokable substances, such as tobacco (AKA: Coolie), marijuana or hashish (see previous section), PCP (AKA: Space Dust), opium, or amphetamines.

How It's Used

Most people go for the coke high by snorting, that is, by inhaling cocaine hydrochloride into the nose. Some users dissolve this substance in water and inject it. Others smoke crack.

The high from snorting begins within three to five minutes, peaks at 20 to 30 minutes, and lasts 40 to 50 minutes overall. For those who shoot, the "rush" hits within a few seconds and peaks within two to three minutes. Smoking delivers great quantities of cocaine—from lungs to blood to brain—within seconds, providing a rush that is similar to shooting up. Those with a needle habit might shoot up every 10 to 20 minutes for hours on end, and dedicated "crack stars" might toke up every five to 10 minutes for hours. Users refer to their continued, repetitive use over long periods of time as "missions" or "runs."

Popularity

Between 9% and 11% of Americans have tried cocaine. About 1.9% have used it within the past year, and 0.8% have used it within the past month. That's almost 1.8 million people who are current users.

When asked specifically about crack, about 2.2% of Americans say they've tried it. About 0.6% have used it within the past year, and 0.3% have used it within the past month. That's equivalent to about 668,000 current users.

The Joy of It

Cocaine acts as a stimulant. It exhilarates. It brings on feelings of intense pleasure and euphoria. It wakes us up.

When high, we feel full of energy and confidence. Often we become more talkative, more physically active, or both. Cocaine depresses our appetite while heightening our sense of potency. We might feel more potent sexually, physically, or mentally.

When injecting cocaine, different people get different effects. Some might feel nauseous or experience upset stomach. Others might experience physical or even mental distress. Yet, almost universally, any unpleasant side effects will give way to an overpowering high or "rush." Users variously describe this rush as "sheer pleasure," "a total body orgasm," or "body electrification." Crack smokers report the same kind of riveting sensations from the rush. However, on a single run each successive shot or toke becomes less electrifying. Nevertheless, the user remembers that initial blast and keeps trying to replicate it. This is called "chasing the high."

In his 1967 book *Pimp: The Story of My Life,* "Iceberg Slim" described the rush from cocaine injection as follows:

"I shivered when it daggered in. . . . I saw the blood-streaked liquid draining into me. It was like a ton of nitro exploded inside me. My ticker went berserk. I could feel clawing up my throat. It was like I had a million 'swipes' in every pore from head to toe. It was like they were all popping off together in a nerve-shredding climax.

"I was quivering like a joker in the hot seat at the first jolt. I tried to open my talc-dry mouth. I couldn't. I was paralyzed. I could feel a hot ball of puke racing up from my careening guts. I saw the green, stinking puke rope arch into the black mouth of the waste basket. . . .

"I felt like the top of my skull had been crushed in. It was like I had been blown apart and all that was left were my eyes. Then tiny prickly feet of ecstasy started dancing through me. I heard melodious bells tolling softly inside my skull.

"I looked down at my hands and thighs. A thrill shot through me. Surely they were the most beautiful in the Universe. I felt a superman's surge of power."

The Problems It Causes

Heart problems. Cocaine increases the blood pressure and heart rate in every user. In many users, it causes irregular heartbeat (arrhythmia).

Lung problems. Cocaine dilates the bronchioles (the breathing tubes in the lungs). In fact, this action can offer temporary relief of asthma symptoms. However, symptoms of asthma increase when coming off cocaine, even among people who don't have asthma. In other words, the bronchioles become more restricted than usual, and breathing becomes strained.

If you smoke crack, your lungs take an extra hard hit because of the direct effects of the smoke. Some symptoms include constant hacking cough, bronchitis, coughing up blood (hemoptysis), and excessive fluid in the lungs (pulmonary edema). Also, recent studies have linked crack smoking with lung cancer.

Nose and throat problems. If you snort coke, your chances of getting nose and throat problems increase significantly. Symptoms include inflammation of the lining of the nose (rhinitis), nasal bleeding, thinning of the lining of the nasal passages (nasal mucosa atrophy), inflammation of the sinuses (sinusitis), hoarseness, and difficulty swallowing.

Danger of infection. If you shoot up coke, you run the risk of various infections. These include infections on the skin (abscesses) or infections under the skin (cellulitis) at injection sites, infection of the liver (hepatitis B), infection of the heart valves (bacterial endocarditis), AIDS, and the spread of infection throughout the body (sepsis).

Gastrointestinal problems. Cocaine raises the blood sugar by causing the liver to convert glycogen into glucose. Over a long period of time, this can lead to malfunction of the liver or pancreas. The pancreas produces insulin to regulate blood sugar. In every user, cocaine depresses the appetite, which over time can lead to weight loss. Coke also depletes the body's store of vitamins, causing various vitamin deficiencies. On using, it often causes dry mouth and in some users causes vomiting or diarrhea.

Sexual dysfunction. When injected or smoked, cocaine can produce a spontaneous ejaculation. However, having sex while high is generally more difficult. Men find it hard to maintain an erection. Women typically cannot reach orgasm.

Anxiety. Prolonged use of coke can lead to anxiety. Those who are affected become nervous, fidgety, and tense. Also this can generalize. We can experience the symptoms of anxiety long after we stop using.

Depression. Every time we come off cocaine, we get depressed. The longer the run and the more we used on the run, the deeper our depression becomes. It also generalizes. We can experience depression for months, even years, after breaking a long-term cocaine addiction. As part of our depression, we often find that nothing feels pleasurable anymore. That's why, during a bout of depression, our coke cravings are highest. We can remember how much pleasure we felt when using. But in recovery, we gradually experience greater and greater pleasure in our lives as our brain chemistry slowly returns to normal.

Mental illness. Cocaine can precipitate a mental illness or can cause us to appear mentally ill for a period of time. Coke commonly fills us with paranoia. We might begin thinking that someone's at the door or at the window. We think we hear them. We might start looking out the curtains every few seconds. Some of us experience paranoid fears after just two hits of crack or two shots of coke. But the longer the run, the more likely we are to get paranoid fears, and the worse the fears become. They usually go away within a few days after we stop using. However, a small percentage of long-term heavy users fall into a paranoid psychosis that remains for life. Aside from delusions (such as the idea that "people are out to get me"), users can also hallucinate. These can be visual (seeing things that aren't there), auditory (hearing things), or tactile (feeling things). One type of tactile hallucination induced by cocaine is sometimes called "coke bugs," the feeling that bugs are crawling on your skin.

Seizure and stroke. Research proves that cocaine use causes seizures in some people and strokes in others. Although grievous, these side effects are rare, occurring in a small percentage of people.

Danger of overdose. In significantly high doses, cocaine can kill in one of two ways: by causing heart attack or by causing respiratory failure. What's a significantly high dose? Some experts figure the fatal dose of
cocaine to be about one gram. This might be enough to
take the life of a newcomer, but there are reports of
heavy users having survived more than 20 grams.

Occasionally, a famous person dies of cocaine
overdose, someone such as Len Bias, who makes the
front page and becomes the lead story on the television news. Yet for every well-publicized cocaine
death, there are hundreds more about which we never
hear. It does happen, but, compared to overdose
deaths from other substances such as heroin, death
from cocaine overdose is relatively rare.

Withdrawal

When coming off coke, you can expect to be tired, depressed, and hungry. You might also have little patience, become easily irritated, or have a negative outlook on life.

You'll almost certainly feel intense cravings for
more substance. The longer and heavier your use,
the longer it'll take these cravings to go away. In recovery, cravings can remain intense for months.
Gradually, the intensity and frequency of cravings
decrease, but even years later a craving might occasionally pop up.

HALLUCINOGENS

People have used hallucinogens for millennia. For one
thing, they're everywhere. Mind-bending biochemicals can be found in thousands of plant species all

over the world and even in some animals. For another thing, they bring on a powerful "consciousness-expanding" experience. People using them see the world in a different way. Reality becomes more multivaried or more profound than what we imagined. Throughout human history, people of different cultures have adopted various, locally available hallucinogens for healing or spiritual purposes.

In addition to the naturally occurring hallucinogens, you can now find many chemically developed synthetics. As you'll soon see, there's a veritable alphabet soup of these new "designer hallucinogens."

Options

Lysergic acid diethylamide (LSD). This product is synthesized from chemical derivatives of a fungus, ergot, that grows on rye and other grains. Usual doses on the street vary from 100 to 700 micrograms (one microgram is a millionth of a gram). One ounce of LSD provides about 300,000 doses. AKA: Acid, Blotter Acid, Big D, Microdot, Yellow Sunshine, Trips, Purple Haze, Window Pane.

Psilocybin. This is the psychoactive ingredient of various species of mushrooms commonly found in Central America and in the warmer climates of the United States. Anywhere from four to 12 mushrooms equal one trip. The hallucinogenic alkaloid 4-hydroxy-dimethyltryptamine (psilocybin) can also be synthesized in a lab. AKA: Magic Mushrooms, Sacred Mushrooms, Shrooms, Silly Putty.

Mescaline. This psychoactive substance occurs naturally in the cactus peyote. People most commonly use the tops of the plant, known as the "buttons." Laboratory enthusiasts have been able to extract the hallucinogenic alkaloid from the peyote cactus and sell it in capsule form. AKA: Mesc, Mescal, Big Chief, Buttons, Moon, P, Peyote.

Morning glory seeds. The seeds of three species of morning glory (trade names: Heavenly Blues, Flying Saucers, Pearly Gates) contain amides of lysergic acid that produce a high similar to that of LSD. It takes about 300 seeds to produce effects similar to 200 to 300 micrograms of LSD.

DMT, 5-MeO-DMT, DET, AET. Dimethyltryptamine (DMT) can be found in a variety of plants worldwide. Many South American tribes make it into a snuff called yopa or cohoba. DMT has also been synthesized and is most often available in the United States as a pure compound (AKA: Businessman's Special or Businessman's High, both terms deriving from the relative short duration of the trip, about 45 minutes, which could easily fit a businessman's scheduled lunch hour). A similar compound, 5-methoxy-dimethyltryptamine (5-MeO-DMT), is found in the skin of some toads and in the seeds of various trees. It has been used for centuries by indigenous peoples and recently found its way onto the streets. Some analogs (compounds with similar chemical structure) have similar hallucinogenic properties. These include diethyltryptamine (DET) and alpha-ethyltryptamine (AET).

Amphetamine-based hallucinogens. Producers with a little chemical savvy have synthesized many variations of mescaline and amphetamine compounds. The first of these to hit the streets in force was DOM (4-methyl-2, 5-dimethoxyamphetamine). This became known in the 1970s as STP ("Scientifically Treated Petroleum"), after a brand name of motor oil additive, but the initials quickly came to stand for the words "Serenity, Tranquility, and Peace" or "Street Trucking People." Other combinations include MDA (methylenedioxyamphetamine), DOB (4-

bromo-2, 5-dimethoxyamphetamine), DMA (dimeth-oxyamphetamine), TMA (trimethoxyamphetamine), MDMA (methylenedioxymethamphetamine), and MDEA (methylenedioxyethylamphetamine). AKA for MDMA: Ecstasy, X, XTC, Love Drug, M & M, Adam. AKA for MDEA: Eve.

Belladonna alkaloids. A large group of "organic" hallucinogens derive from a family of plants (Solanaceae) that contains about 3,000 members. These include species of mandrake, henbane, and belladonna. Some of the belladonna alkaloids, such as atropine, act as poisons and are lethal in high doses; other alkaloids, such as scopolamine, act as hallucinogens. The most common plant on the U.S. scene is *Datura stramonium,* known variously as jimsonweed, stinkweed, thorn apple, and devil's apple.

Combinations. Some users will smoke marijuana with hallucinogens to calm themselves or to boost the hallucinogenic effect. Some will use sedatives to slow things down or to calm an otherwise rocky trip. A few users will combine hallucinogens with stimulants such as cocaine, crack, or amphetamines. AKA for combining LSD and crack: Sheet Rocking.

How They're Used

Most commonly, people take hallucinogens orally. LSD is swallowed in tablets, tiny squares of gelatin (called "window pane"), or premeasured drops on blotter paper. Users trip on psilocybin by eating the mushrooms and on mescaline by eating the dried cactus buttons or by taking either of these chemicals in tablet or capsule form. Some users take mescaline by first soaking the buttons in water and then drinking the liquid. Morning glory trippers usually grind the seeds into a flour and swallow them with water or soak the flour in water for a period of time and then drink it. The leaves and seeds of jimsonweed and other plants bearing belladonna alkaloids can be eaten directly. Some users make a tea from these plants and drink that. The high from this group of substances lasts from six to 12 hours, with LSD and mescaline falling on the high end (10 to 12 hours) and morning glory seeds on the low end (six to eight hours).

The tryptamines (DMT, DET, AET, and 5-MeO-DMT) are most often sniffed or smoked. When taken orally, these compounds metabolize too fast to produce a psychoactive effect—except for 5-MeO-DMT, which can be milked from the glands of the toads and ingested. The trip duration for all these is brief: a half hour to an hour and a half.

Users commonly take the mescaline-like amphetamines orally, in tablet form, although sometimes they're snorted. The high from this group of drugs typically lasts six to eight hours.

Popularity

About 9.7% of Americans have tried hallucinogens. About 1.7% have used one of the hallucinogens within the past year, and 0.6% have used one within the past month. That's more than 1,300,000 people who have used hallucinogens within the past month. Of these current users, 454,000 were aged 12 to 17, and 627,000 were aged 18 to 25.

The Joy of It

The experiences that people get from hallucinogens vary more than what people get from any other class of drugs. Even one person using the same hallucinogen can have vastly different experiences with each use.

The types of experiences that a given person will have depends on *set* and *setting*. Set refers to the person—to what the person expects to get out of the trip. It also refers to the person's mood at the outset—to his or her previous experiences while tripping—and to personality; for example, whether the person is introverted or extroverted, intellectual or emotional, was subjected to childhood trauma or had a carefree childhood. Setting refers to the external details—whom the person is with, where the person is, and what's going on in the immediate environment. Tripping in a crowded bar with friends has an entirely different feel to it than tripping quietly alone in one's room.

The fun derived from hallucinogens comes primarily from the profound changes that it causes in our perceptions and moods. However, because each trip is so unpredictable, some users get top jollies simply by hopping a wild ride into the realm of the unexpected.

The effects from different hallucinogens vary. All produce vast changes in perception or mood. However, some are more perception or mind oriented, such as LSD, psilocybin, mescaline, morning glory seeds, and the tryptamine group; others are more mood or body oriented, such as the amphetamine-based hallucinogens (MDMA became known as Ecstasy or the Love Drug for good reason) and the belladonna alkaloids.

All hallucinogens distort our perception of time. Time appears to slow down. A moment can become an eternity. And all hallucinogens distort our perception of space. Boundaries appear to dissolve. Edges become fuzzy. When we're observing a tree against a background of sky, the tree becomes sky, and the sky blends into the tree. The two can even fuse together as one. Sometimes everything around us can appear to be pulsating or vibrating, one thing turning into another. The small becomes large, the large small. Shapes can magically change. Sounds can undulate so deep within us that we experience them in the belly. We can hug the earth and actually feel it rumbling.

In addition, hallucinogens have the power to dissolve the ego. The boundary between self and others disappears. The boundary between self and world disappears. Sometimes we can have an out-of-body experience (OOB). We might feel as if we left our body and that we're somewhere else in the room watching what we're doing. Some of us even imagine that we're traveling astrally during an OOB and going elsewhere in the universe. And sometimes, we imagine that we've actually met with God or Buddha or Jesus or some other key spiritual figure.

Indeed, tearing down the walls of the ego often becomes a spiritual experience. It can leave us feeling more connected with "the whole"—with God, with others, or with the world around us. It feels as if we're opening ourselves to something greater, something more than what's inside. This occurs in a common hallucination. When tripping, many imagine themselves as a bud on a lush, leafy stem that opens into a brilliant flower.

Hallucinogens, like marijuana, bring on two types of high: intellectual (head trip) or emotional (body trip). Which type you get depends on set and setting and the particular hallucinogen you use.

On a head trip, we experience heightened awareness. Everything about the world becomes more vivid, more ecstatic. The senses become paramount. The world becomes extravagant. We can see, hear, taste, touch, and smell in more wondrous detail than we've ever known.

On a body trip, we experience a deeper sense of connection with ourselves or others. We feel love. We might imagine that we become love. We begin to understand others or ourselves as we never have before. We might experience our feelings as all-encompassing. We feel whole, complete. We might enjoy sex as a beautiful spiritual union.

The Problems It Causes

Physical. For LSD, psilocybin, mescaline, and morning glory seeds, the problems from physical side effects include some nausea; increased body temperature, heart rate, and blood pressure; some muscle weakness or tremor; and occasionally diarrhea. The tryptamines lead to similar problems but in addition cause greater muscle weakness, sometimes to the point of temporary paralysis. The amphetamine-based hallucinogens and the belladonna alkaloids bring about the greatest physical dangers. They cause severe changes in heart rate, breathing, and body temperature. In addition, the amphetamine group causes amphetamine-like hyperactivity, and at least one of this group, MDMA, often causes users to clench their teeth.

Brain damage. Studies show that MDMA causes irreversible damage to nerve cell endings, which contain serotonin in their storage vesicles. Other amphetamine-based hallucinogens may cause this serious problem as well. Currently, more research is needed to know for sure.

Bad trips. A trip can be deep, frightening, dark or light, euphoric, and airy. It can even change from one to the other quickly. Nonetheless, some users accept bad trips, believing them to be enlightening. Even venturing into dark spaces can bring insight.

However, other users find bad trips a reason to quit using hallucinogens. A trip might have caused fears that are too intense to bear. Of course, tripping does bring unconscious memories into full awareness, and because of this a trip can produce deep psychic pain. It can bring forth memories of childhood trauma in all-too-vivid detail.

Indeed, any feelings can explode into difficulties. A feeling of sadness can bring us to our knees in tears, something disgusting can become outrageously gross, and a simple fear can transform itself into our worst nightmare.

A trip can also induce panic attacks. Another person, an object, or the whole world can take on such a frightening, eerie air that it can scare us half to death. We might imagine ourselves being killed in some frightening way, such as being buried alive. When in a crowd, we might imagine that each person is a poisonous snake attempting to strike at us. We might imagine a shadow on the wall to be a roaring locomotive heading straight at us.

Loss of ego. Although ego dissolution can be enlightening to some, it can be psychologically damaging to others. The ego is a protective device. It helps define who we are. When it is dissolved, we become vulnerable. We can feel completely lost. Our sense of direction in life—our ability to pursue goals—can be shattered; this happens to a significant percentage of users. Although the ego will never be the same, it will heal reasonably well after a few months to a year or so of abstinence.

Flashbacks. Also called post-hallucinogenic perceptual disorder (PHPD), flashbacks refer to the recurrence of a hallucinogenic experience at a time when you're not taking the drug. It can be one of two things:

a memory of something that happened while you were tripping or a brief period during which you perceive things as if you were tripping. Flashbacks last anywhere from a few seconds to 10 minutes or more. They're unpredictable and can be an annoying inconvenience because, when they occur, they're so completely distracting.

A memory flashback is usually triggered by a person, an object, or an event that reminds you of something that occurred while tripping. This trigger can bring forth an entire memory sequence, complete with the vivid detail, hallucinations, or feelings that you experienced in the original scene.

A perceptual flashback might have you experiencing altered visual images, the blending of images and sounds, a pulsating visual field, fuzzy images, a tingling sensation on the skin, or tracers (trails of light). Perceptual flashbacks can occur because the brain has actually been changed by the hallucinogenic drug. Research on people who had recently used LSD showed that their visual systems continued to respond to stimuli after the stimuli had been removed. The change was slight but measurable. This suggests that LSD might alter the brain's perceptual hardware, at least for a period of time.

About 60% of heavy LSD users (those who've tripped more than 20 times) report that they've experienced some amount of flashbacks. About 40% of heavy users report none.

Flashbacks diminish over time after a user is abstinent. They usually disappear after a few months, although they persist in some people for more than a year.

Psychosis. Many researchers in the 1960s and 1970s called hallucinogens "psychotomimetic" drugs because they mimicked a psychotic state in those who used them. For one thing, hallucinogens cause hallucinations in most users. For another, they make many users feel split off from reality. These are two hallmark symptoms of the psychosis schizophrenia. Because of this, you would think that hallucinogens would make many people psychotic, but hallucinogens trigger psychosis in only a small percentage of users (0.1% to 0.5%). Still, this is significant, especially if you're one of the users who was affected this way.

Harm from accidents. Occasionally, people will hurt themselves while tripping. Usually, this stems from users' hallucinations or errors of judgment. Some users have jumped out of windows or off roofs fully thinking that they can fly. Some have hurt themselves when escaping from hallucinated monsters. Some have made mistakes while driving. Every so often, someone dies from a hallucinogen-induced accident.

Danger of overdose. Most of the hallucinogens are safe in high doses, but a few can be toxic. Deaths due to cardiac arrest have occurred in people using MDMA and have been recorded in users of MDEA. The use of 5-MeO-DMT can also kill. The skin of a single toad contains enough of this substance to be fatal. Finally, thousands of deaths throughout history can be attributed to belladonna poisoning. The belladonna alkaloids are probably the most dangerous of the hallucinogens because the dose that causes the desired effects—hallucinations and mild delirium—is very near the lethal dose.

Withdrawal

For a couple of days after a trip, a user can feel worn out and become reflective or contemplative. Other than this short period of recuperation, there is no significant withdrawal syndrome for the hallucinogens.

INHALANTS

Through the wizardry of modern chemical science, we now have available dozens of substances that produce psychoactive vapors. There's nothing natural here. These substances are purely the product of industry. Among the inhalants are three remarkably different types of substances: nitrous oxide and other anesthetic gases, nitrites, and solvents and aerosols.

Options

Nitrous oxide and other anesthetic gases. Nitrous oxide, also known as laughing gas, has a medical use as a dental anesthetic. It's also used as the propellant in whipped-cream containers. It comes in small metal cylinders called "whippets" by those in the drug culture. Some users inhale this gas from balloons or from special pipes called "buzz bombs." Other anesthetic gases that people sometimes abuse are ether, chloroform, and halothane. However, none of these is as common on the street.

Nitrites. The nitrites are yellow, flammable liquids that have a fruity odor. The best known of these, amyl nitrite, can be obtained by prescription for alleviating heart pain (angina). It comes in ampoules that, when broken, release the fumes (AKA: Poppers, Snappers, Amies, Pearls). Other nitrites include butyl nitrite (which until 1995 was sold legally as room deodorizers and liquid incense) and isobutyl nitrite. AKA for butyl nitrite: Rush, Kick, Locker Room, Locker Popper, Jock Aroma, Satan's Scent, Toilet Water. AKA for isobutyl nitrite: Bolt, Bullets, Climax.

Solvents and aerosols. This group includes gasoline, lighter fluid, glues, refrigerants, paint, lacquers, paint thinners, paint sprays, degreasers, cleaning solutions, correction fluids, felt-tip marker fluid, fabric protector sprays, and hair or deodorant sprays. Users can inhale these chemicals directly or by using a soaked rag. Another method involves saturating a cotton ball or rag, placing it in a paper or plastic bag, and inhaling the contents. This is called "bagging." AKA for breathing solvents and aerosols: Huffing.

How They're Used

All these substances are inhaled through the nose or mouth. Users simply breathe the fumes.

Each substance in this category produces a brief high—lasting from two to five minutes with each inhalation. A deeper high, to the point of delirium or intoxication, comes from continuous inhalation over a short period of time. Nevertheless, once the user stops inhaling, the high begins to fade and usually ends within five minutes for nitrites and gaseous anesthetics and within 10 to 20 minutes for solvents and aerosols.

Popularity

About 5.6% of Americans have used one or more of the inhalants at some time in their lives. About 1.1% have used one or more during the past year, and 0.4% have used within the past month. That's about 961,000 current users. Of these, 391,000 were aged 12 to 17, and 289,000 were aged 18 to 25.

The Joy of It

Nitrous oxide and the gaseous anesthetics. Nitrous oxide is the mildest of the gaseous anesthetics. It reduces pain and increases the sense of euphoria. It can also lower inhibitions while increasing mental exhilaration, so things often seem funnier than usual. At higher concentrations, it causes drowsiness. The other gaseous anesthetics produce these effects as well but at higher concentrations cause major sedation.

Nitrites. The nitrites relax the smooth muscles of the body—those that control blood vessels, the bladder, the anus, and other tissues. Users often feel as if their bodies go limp. They might also feel light-headed or faint. Indeed, after popping, some users collapse into a giddy heap on the floor.

Because the nitrites relax the muscles that regulate the blood vessels, they produce an increased heart rate along with a drop in blood pressure. Most users feel sensations of pleasure and warmth, and some take nitrites to boost the pleasure of sex. Some users report that when they're high they feel that their orgasms last longer. The nitrites gained favor among gay men for this reason and for the added reason that these drugs relax the anal sphincter muscle, making penetration easier.

Solvents and aerosols. This group of chemicals produces an intoxication similar to that of alcohol. Users experience reduced inhibitions, increased mental energy or exhilaration, and feelings of physical calm. Continued huffing in a single session leads to drowsiness, numbness, and even unconsciousness. Continued use can also cause dizziness, disorientation, delusions, and hallucinations. Users might "see" shooting stars, ghosts, or angels and "hear" deafening explosions, unusual voices, or music from the center of the universe. Some of the reported delusions include feeling as if you can fly, feeling as if you're a supremely powerful hero or villain, or feeling as if you can walk through walls.

The Problems It Causes

Nitrous oxide. Users sometimes experience injuries to the mouth, trachea, or lungs because of the cooling effects of expanding gas. Users also run the risk of death by asphyxiation if they don't ensure a supply of oxygen-rich air. This happens occasionally when someone falls into unconsciousness and breathes only nitrous oxide. Long-term users have problems with vitamin B12 deficiency. Nitrous oxide inactivates B12, which causes the destruction of nerve fibers (neuropathy). Physical symptoms of this damage include weakness, tingling sensations, decreased sense of touch, abnormalities in gait, decreased ankle and knee reflexes, and bladder and bowel dysfunction. Psychological symptoms include loss of memory, depression, confusion, and delirium.

Nitrites. Side effects of using nitrites include headaches, flushing of the skin, cold sweats, dizziness, and the potential to drop briefly into unconsciousness. Some users get crusty lesions on the skin around the mouth, nose, penis, and scrotum. Some users get skin rashes or irritations of the throat and eyes. Nitrites also cause a decrease in the blood's ability to carry oxygen (methemoglobinemia). This can be serious enough to cause coma or death. The early signs of methemoglobinemia are breathlessness combined with the lips, tongue, and hands turning blue. This condition becomes most serious when nitrites have been swallowed rather than inhaled.

Solvents and aerosols. Among all the drugs of abuse, solvents and aerosols might be the most dangerous. Once inside the body, these chemicals wreak destruction. They cause serious damage to the liver, kidneys, muscles, gastrointestinal system, and cardiovascular system and to the brain and nervous system. In long-term moderate users and short-term heavy users, damage to the kidneys, the nervous system, and the brain can be irreversible.

Studies show that these chemicals have caused thousands of deaths. The term "sudden sniffing death" (SSD) refers to death from cardiac arrest. Inhaling coolants (such as freon), propellants from hair spray or spray paint, and fuel gases (such as butane and propane) often lead to heart arrhythmias that can end in cardiac arrest. About 50% of all inhalant deaths are SSDs. Another significant percentage of sniffers die from suffocation. This occurs when a user becomes unconscious and falls on a rag containing one of the solvents or becomes unconscious when huffing from a plastic bag placed over the head. A small percentage who use aerosol products have died from freezing of the airways (laryngospasm). Another small percentage of sniffers and huffers have died from inhalation of vomit after falling into an unconscious or a semiconscious state. A large percentage of deaths from inhalant use can be attributed to accidents. One broad-based study of 1,239 inhalant deaths showed that 26% were due to accidents.

Withdrawal

There's no documented abstinence syndrome for nitrous oxide and the nitrites. Some long-term heavy users of solvents and aerosols experience a withdrawal syndrome that includes stomach cramps, chills, hallucinations, and delirium tremens (DTs). However, this syndrome is rare.

HEROIN, OPIATES, AND THE ANALGESICS

Heroin and the opiates derive from the poppy plant, *Papaver somniferum*, which displays a beautiful flower when in full bloom. Opium is the sticky, tarry sub-stance produced within this plant's seed pod.

For the past 6,000 years, the opium poppy has been cultivated for use in various medicinal prepara-tions. Some of the earliest medicinals from this plant were probably in the form of teas. We have evidence that people began smoking opium about 3,000 years ago in areas of Asia, Egypt, and Europe. In the Middle Ages, a preparation of opium called laudanum gained popularity in Europe. In 1803 the psychoactive sub-stance morphine was isolated from an opium base, and in 1898 the semisynthetic heroin was refined from morphine.

The opiates have many medical uses, and many have been used for years as painkillers (analgesics). Also, because they cause respiratory depression and constipation, various preparations have been used as cough suppressants or antidiarrheals. To meet medical demands each year, the U.S. pharmaceutical industry imports more than 500 tons of opium or its equiva-lent in poppy straw concentrate for the production of prescription opiates.

Today we have dozens of opiates. Some, such as heroin, are produced and sold illegally; others are pro-duced legally but find their way into illegal markets on the streets. The opiates fall into three general cate-gories: naturally occurring (opium, morphine, codeine, and thebaine), semisynthetic (heroin, hydromorphone, oxycodone, hydrocodone, and buprenorphine), and synthetic (meperidine, methadone, LAAM, dextro-propoxyphene, fentanyl, and pentazocine).

Options

Opium. This product is made from the thick, glue-like liquid that oozes from the plant's seed pod. Producers dry it into a ball (gum opium) or pound it into a powder (opium powder). Opium is the active ingredient in various medicines used for the treatment of diarrhea (trade names: Paregoric, Parepectolin, Donnagel-PG). It's also available in a couple of pain remedies (trade names: Pantopon, B&O Supprettes). AKA: O, Big O, Zero, Dreams, Gem, Hop, Tar, Skee, Toys, Chinese Molasses, Gong, Black Stuff, Black Pills. AKA for paregoric: Blue Velvet.

Morphine. This substance was named after Morpheus, the Greek god of dreams who was often depicted with a handful of opium poppies. Morphine is the principal psychoactive chemical in opium, ranging in concentrations from 4% to 21%. It is probably the most effective painkiller (analgesic) known to humans. In fact, it provides a standard against which new analgesics are measured. Morphine is prescribed mainly for the treatment of pain and sometimes as an adjunct to anesthesia. Trade names: Morphine Sulphate, Morphine Sulphate Injection, MS Contin, Oramorph SR, Duramorph, Roxanol. AKA: M, Morph, M.S., Dreamer, Miss Emma.

Codeine. This psychoactive alkaloid occurs in opium in concentrations ranging from 0.7% to 2.5%. Compared to morphine, it produces less sedation and respiratory depression and less analgesia. It is prescribed for relief of moderate pain or as an effective cough suppressant. Codeine has become the most widely used naturally occurring opiate in medical treatment in the world. Trade names: Codeine Phosphate Injection, Acetaminophen with Codeine, Aspirin with Codeine, Fiorinal with Codeine, Phenaphen with Codeine, Synalgos, Tylenol with Codeine, Robitussin AC, Empirin with Codeine. AKA: Schoolboys, Pops.

Thebaine. This chemical occurs in small quantities in opium. It's similar chemically to morphine and codeine but has stimulant rather than depressant effects. Thebaine has no therapeutic value but is the precursor to a variety of other psychoactive or therapeutic compounds. These include hydrocodone, oxycodone, oxymorphone, nalbuphine, naloxone, naltrexone, and buprenorphine.

Heroin. This drug was first synthesized from morphine in 1898 by the Bayer Company in Germany. It got its name from the German *heroisch,* which means "powerful." This semisynthetic enters the brain more quickly than morphine because chemically it's more soluble in fat. Once in the brain, it turns back into morphine. Heroin is most commonly available in powder form. Its color varies from pure white to dark brown. Sellers package it by the "bag," each of which contains one dose equal to about 100 milligrams. In recent years, the purity of heroin on the street has improved. In 1980, the national average purity of heroin was 3.6%. In 1993, it was 37%. Another form of heroin known as "black tar" has hit the streets in recent years. Some varieties are gummy and sticky, whereas others are as hard as coal. It ranges in color from brown to black. This product hails from Mexico, where crude processing methods prevail, thus the dark color. Its purity ranges from 20% to 80%. AKA: H, Big H, Horse, Smack, White Lady, White Stuff, Junk, Dope, Mojo, Downtown, Brown, Mexican Brown, Mud.

Hydromorphone. This semisynthetic opiate has an analgesic potency two to eight times that of morphine. Trade names: Dilaudid, Dilaudid-HP Injection, Hydromorphone Hydrochloride. AKA: D, Dilly, Fours, Lords.

Hydrocodone. This semisynthetic opiate works as an analgesic and as a cough remedy (antitussive). Trade names: Anexsia, Hycodan, Hycomine, Lorcet, Lortab, Tussionex, Vicodin.

Oxycodone. This substance is more potent than codeine and more addictive. Trade names: Percodan, Percocet, Tylox.

Meperidine. Compared to morphine, this synthetic opiate produces similar analgesia but has a shorter duration of action and reduced antitussive and antidiarrheal effects. Trade name: Demerol.

Fentanyl. This synthetic opiate acts as a highly potent form of heroin. It has medical uses as an analgesic and as an anesthetic (trade name for anesthetic fentanyl: Sublimaze). At least 12 analogs of this drug have been created. Some have medical uses as analgesics, such as alfentyl (trade name: Alfenta) and sufentanil (trade name: Sufenta). Drug marketers have produced numerous fentanyls that are sold on the street. Some of these are 100 times more potent than street-quality heroin. AKA: China White, Tango and Cash.

Pentazocine. This synthetic provides mild analgesia. Trade names: Talwin, Talacin.

Methadone and related synthetics. Methadone acts like heroin or morphine but doesn't resemble the opiates in chemical form. Medically, it's used in heroin detoxification and maintenance programs. Methadone's effects last longer than heroin's—up to 24 hours—so it's ideal for once-a-day maintenance doses (AKA: Dollies, Dolls, Wafers, Ten-Eight-Twenty). A chemical cousin to methadone, levo-al-phacetylmethadol (LAAM) produces similar effects to methadone but lasts even longer. In 1994 this drug was approved as an alternative treatment for narcotics addiction (trade name: ORLAAM). Currently, researchers are testing yet another drug, the semisynthetic opiate buprenorphine, for use in treatment of narcotics addiction (trade name: Buprenex). Another relative of methadone, propoxyphene, acts as a weak analgesic and is not much stronger than aspirin (trade names: Darvon-N, Darvon Compound-65, Darvocet-N 100, Wygesic). AKA: Pinks-and-Greys.

Other synthetics. This group includes alphaprodine (trade name: Nisentil), which is prescribed for pain; diphenoxylate (Lomotil) for diarrhea; levorphanol (Levo-Dromoran) for pain; loperamide (Immodium) for diarrhea; buteorphanol (Stadol) for pain; and nalbuphine (Nubain) for pain.

Combinations. Users have combined this group of drugs with many other substances. Some of the more popular combinations (along with the street names for each) include heroin and cocaine (Speedball, Whizz Bang, Dynamite, Murder One), heroin and tobacco (Duster), heroin and marijuana (Atom Bomb, A-Bomb), heroin or another opiate with amphetamines, opium with marijuana (O.J.), Talwin with the antihistamine pyribenzamine (T's and Blues).

How They're Used

A large percentage of heroin users go for the high by injection, either intravenously ("mainlining"), subcutaneously ("skin popping"), or intramuscularly. As the purity of heroin has increased, however, more occasional users, called "chippers," have entered dreamland by snorting or smoking the powder. Opium users almost always smoke the substance.

Hardcore heroin addicts will seek most any analgesic when the smack supply runs short. A favorite is Dilaudid. If the substance comes in tablet form, as Dilaudid does, users will often grind it into powder, dissolve it in water, and shoot it. Otherwise, both chippers and hardcore addicts will take analgesics the way they were intended, that is, orally in tablets, capsules, or liquid preparations.

The high from most of the opiates lasts from two to six hours. However, at one extreme fentanyl lasts only an hour or so, and at the other LAAM lasts a couple of days. The high from fentanyl injection is the quickest of all the analgesics to reach peak levels in the brain (two to four seconds). Heroin is slower, taking a couple of minutes, and morphine takes about five minutes. The high from snorting heroin takes even longer to reach peak levels, and anyone who takes analgesics orally must wait the longest for the high to hit, about a half hour or so.

Researchers find two patterns of abuse. In one pattern, users start on the streets with illicit opiates. These users start as chippers, some of whom graduate to greater and greater use and some of whom don't. Typically, they begin by snorting, smoking, pill popping, or drinking liquid preparations such as cough syrups or Paragoric. Those who graduate go to skin popping or mainlining. In the other pattern, users get started on analgesics in a medical setting and, over a period of time, develop "a habit." They become addicted to their prescribed medication. Typically, these users begin "doctor shopping." They bounce from doctor to doctor seeking scripts for painkillers, often faking symptoms with the premeditated poise of great actors and actresses. Many who follow this pattern of addiction will, at some point, begin seeking illicit opiates on the street.

Popularity

About 5.5% of Americans have used illicit analgesics. About 2.1% have used illicit analgesics within the past year, and about 0.9% have used them within the past month. That's about 1.9 million current users.

About 2.5 million Americans have used heroin at some time in their lives. About 455,000 have used it within the past year.

The Joy of It

When we take opiates, it's as if Morpheus enters our very being. Everything becomes dream-like. Our cares and troubles float away. Our eyelids, like those of the meditating Buddha, rest serenely in a half-closed position. We feel comfortable. We become drowsy and sleepy, and sometimes we nod off into our very own slumberland. We feel as if we've entered a warm, safe place—a place where we're protected, cared for, and tenderly held—a place very much like the womb.

Mainliners get a rush, a climactic sensation that some compare to orgasm. Although this rush resembles the jolt from cocaine or methamphetamine, it's not as powerfully orgasmic. Mainliners also typically experience a period of nausea along with, or just after, the rush. This discomfort is sometimes resolved by dedicating a few minutes to the act of vomiting.

The opiates were originally called "narcotics," a word derived from the Greek *narcotikos*, meaning "benumbing" or "causing sleep." These numbing sensations, the absence of pain, and the warm, dreamy feelings create a powerful attraction for the recreational use of these drugs.

The Problems It Causes

Lung problems. The opiates cause a decrease in breathing rate and depth. In fact, breathing becomes dangerously impaired at higher doses. In addition, if you smoke opiates, you increase your chances of smoke-related lung problems. You might experience hacking cough, bronchitis, and other difficulties.

Gastrointestinal problems. The opiates cause constipation. Many heavy users can't move their bowels for days and sometimes go for even a week or more without any bowel movements. This problem resolves with abstinence.

Sexual dysfunction. Users experience a decreased sexual desire and a decreased ability to perform sexually. Males often can't get an erection (impotence). This problem usually resolves when opiates are discontinued. However, a small percentage who used opiates addictively, and in combination with other substances, report that their impotence continued long after they had quit all the drugs. Female addicts can experience lack of menstrual period (amenorrhea), which resolves when opiates are discontinued.

Malnutrition. Heavy users tend to be malnourished or undernourished. The reason is uncertain. It may happen because heavy users don't attend to the body's need for food or because they spend too much time and energy acquiring more of the drug.

Danger of infection. If you shoot heroin or other opiates, you run the risk of various infections. These include infections on the skin (abscesses) or under the skin (cellulitis) at injection sites, infection of the veins (thrombophlebitis), inflammation of the veins (often caused by injecting particles that were not ground fine enough to completely dissolve), infection of the liver (hepatitis B), infection of the heart valves (endocarditis), AIDS, and brain and lung abscesses.

Danger of overdose. With opiates, the danger of overdose looms large. The problem arises mainly because these drugs depress the respiration. Death from depressed respiration usually occurs within minutes after an injection. The user falls into a coma and never revives.

Usually, overdose occurs after a single injection. It happens because the dose from that injection is higher than the user could tolerate. With street heroin varying in purity from 10% to 80%, this becomes a real problem. Also with fentanyl and its analogs the danger is even greater because of the greater potency of these synthetics. Since fentanyl came on the scene, it has caused many deaths from overdose. Methadone, too, has led to many overdose deaths due to use in non-medical settings. A note on Darvon: It has numerous toxic side effects and, as reported by medical examiners in the United States, is one of the top 10 drugs in causing drug abuse deaths.

Withdrawal

Withdrawal begins with a runny nose, watery eyes, yawning, and sweating. Then you experience chills and goose bumps (where the term "cold turkey" came from), along with flu-like symptoms, including nausea, vomiting, and diarrhea. You also get muscle aches and spasms and the typical leg-kicking response due to leg spasms (which gave rise to the phrase "kicking the habit"). You also feel pains in the muscles and bones. You're unable to sleep. You might feel anxiety, tension, anger, or hostility. Finally, you feel like nothing is enjoyable in life, and you crave opiates.

The physical symptoms peak at two to four days and disappear within seven to 10 days. The mental symptoms—feeling like nothing's enjoyable and the craving of opiates—will continue. In fact, these two symptoms are connected. You know that opiates will take away any bad feelings and make life enjoyable again. You know this at a gut level. It happens in your mind, but it feels as if your whole body craves. These mental symptoms will last a few months at least, maybe even a year or more. However, they continue to diminish in frequency and intensity as long as you remain in recovery.

AMPHETAMINES AND OTHER STIMULANTS

Amphetamines, diet pills, methylphenidate (Ritalin), and phenylpropanolamine are products of the laboratory. All have been synthesized within the past 125 years. Other stimulants that occur naturally in plants have been used by indigenous peoples for thousands of years. These organic stimulants include cathinone, found in the leaves of the khat plant; ephedrine, found in Chinese ephedra shrubs; caffeine, found in coffee beans, tea leaves, cola nuts, and yerba mate; and nicotine, found in tobacco. (Cocaine is also a stimulant and is covered in a separate section in this chapter.)

Options

Amphetamines. Amphetamine (or amphetamine sulfate) was first available as an over-the-counter inhaler in the 1930s. Called the Benzedrine inhaler, it was recommended for treatment of nasal congestion. Benzedrine was later marketed, in the form of a pill, for the treatment of narcolepsy and for "minimal brain dysfunction" (MBD), which is now called "attention deficit hyperactive disorder" (ADHD). Trade name: Benzedrine. AKA: Uppers, Bennies, Peaches, Whites.

Dextroamphetamine (or dextroamphetamine sulfate) is marketed under the trade name Dexedrine

(AKA: Dexies, Co-pilots, Oranges, Footballs). It's also available in combination with amphetamine under the trade name Biphetamine (AKA: Black Beauties, Black Mollies, Blackbirds).

Methamphetamine hydrochloride, the pharmaceutical product, comes in tablet form (trade name: Desoxyn). The methamphetamine appearing on the street is most often the product of clandestine chemical laboratories. It comes in the form of a crystalline powder (AKA: Speed, Crank, Meth, Crystal Meth, Crystal). Operators of clandestine labs have also produced a crystallized version of methamphetamine hydrochloride that can be smoked (AKA: Ice, Quartz).

Methcathinone is the structural analog of methamphetamine and cathinone, the psychoactive stimulant found in the khat plant. This compound is also the product of clandestine labs. AKA: Cat, Khat, Goob, Crank.

Diet pills. Pharmaceutical companies have developed amphetamine congeners (chemicals that are similar in nature) into today's prescription diet pills. They are milder than the amphetamines yet stronger than caffeine. These include (along with trade names): benzphetamine (Didrex), diethylpropion (Tenuate, Tepanil), fenfluramine (Pondimin), mazindol (Mazanor, Sanorex), phendimetrazine (Bontril, Plegine, Prelu-2, Trimstat), phenmetrazine (Preludin), and phentermine (Adipex-P, Ionamin, Fastin).

Methylphenidate. Manufactured under the trade names Ritalin and Methylphenidate Hydrochloride, this synthetic stimulant has a lower potential for abuse than the amphetamines. Although similar in action to the amphetamines, it packs a weaker punch. Currently, this medication is prescribed for ADHD and for the treatment of narcolepsy.

Phenylpropanolamine. This mild stimulant can be found in many prescription and over-the-counter medications. It's a common ingredient, sometimes in combination with caffeine, in over-the-counter diet pills (trade names: Acutrim, Appendrine, Dexatrim, Ordinex). It also appears in various over-the-counter cough, cold, and allergy remedies (trade names: Alka Seltzer Plus, Contac, Coricidin-D, Naldecon, Sinarest).

Khat. For centuries, people in Arabia and East Africa have cultivated the shrub *Catha edulis* for the production of khat. This product consists of the fresh, young leaves of the khat plant. These are chewed to produce a mild stimulant effect. For the full effect, the leaves must be consumed quickly, usually within 48 hours of picking, because the psychoactive stimulant cathinone converts to a significantly milder stimulant (cathine) as the leaves dry.

Ephedrine. This mild stimulant derives from Chinese ephedras. It has been used for centuries in China for the treatment of hay fever, asthma, and nasal congestion. In recent years, this herbal stimulant has become available through legal, over-the-counter markets in the United States.

Caffeine. This psychoactive chemical occurs naturally in many plants all over the world. It's both legal and widely available. Served in coffees, teas, and carbonated soft drinks as well as chocolate and cocoa concoctions, this mild stimulant acts as a social lubricant or "alertness booster" in low doses. In higher doses, it can turn anyone into a nervous wreck. What's a low dose? One to two cups of coffee, two to three cups of tea, or two to three caffeinated sodas per day—a little more if you're younger, a little less if you're older.

But there's a problem. Caffeine is highly addicting. It's not easy to curtail our consumption. We tend to press ourselves to our personal limit, to get that caffeine buzzing deep inside yet managing to hold the high just short of nervous frenzy. However, some of us can't hold it there and repeatedly overconsume, venturing fitfully into the fray of nervous system overstimulation. This is the group of us who become flatout caffeine addicts. It's primarily to this group that other caffeine products appeal, such as over-the-counter caffeine tablets (trade names: NoDoz, Vivarin), diet pills, headache remedies and cold medications, and prescription headache remedies.

Nicotine. This popular, widely available substance acts as a mild stimulant. It might very well be the single most addicting drug in the world. Few people can use it in moderation. For example, not many can limit their smoking to just a couple of cigarettes a week. In fact, more than 90% of people who use this drug use it addictively, and using tobacco addictively can be a major undertaking. Smokers light up a cigarette anywhere from five to 80 times a day and, with each one, draw in anywhere from 15 to 30 lungfuls of smoke. So that's doing anywhere from 75 to 3,200 "hits" a day. What power this drug has to control our behavior!

In one broad-spectrum study, people rated the difficulty they had quitting various drugs. When the scores were averaged, nicotine ranked the highest, beating out alcohol, heroin, cocaine, and all the other drugs of abuse.

(Note: Although the methods in this book will help you quit smoking, the book was not intended for that purpose. The entry for nicotine has been included here so you'll know that it's a mild stimulant and a powerfully addicting drug. We'll revisit nicotine in Chapter 6, "How to Break a Habit," and Chapter 7, "Healing Through Diet.")

Combinations. Some users inject methamphetamine with heroin in a variation of a speedball. Some smoke ice with other smokables: tobacco, marijuana, or opium. Some use amphetamines in combination with cocaine. However, the most typical combination is the upper-downer combo, pairing stimulants with depressants or analgesics or using the stimulants throughout the day and the depressants in the evening to help with sleep.

How They're Used

Amphetamines can be taken orally, snorted, injected, or, in the case of ice, smoked. The effects of amphetamines—especially the two illegally manufactured powders methamphetamine and methcathinone—are similar to that of cocaine, but the high lasts much longer. The amphetamine high lasts four to five hours and the coke high only 15 to 30 minutes.

The pharmaceuticals—diet pills, methylphenidate, and phenylpropanolamine—are almost always taken in their manufactured form: pills, capsules, or liquids. All these drugs create a pick-me-up that lasts a few hours.

It's rare to find fresh khat leaves on U.S. streets, but it's becoming more common to find its psychoactive constituent cathinone. Users usually snort cathinone, although some inject it and some take it orally. Users who go for the herbal stimulant ephedrine usually take it orally in powders or capsules, although many sip it in the form of tea.

People go for the caffeine buzz by pounding cup after cup of coffee, tea, or soda. Heavy users sometimes add various over-the-counter pills and preparations to their menu of caffeine delights.

Popularity

About 4.7% of us have used illicit stimulants at some time in our lives. About 0.9% have used illicit stimulants within the past year, and 0.4% have used within the past month. That's 763,000 who are current users. These figures don't include legally prescribed stimulants, over-the-counter stimulants, and caffeine.

The Joy of It

Stimulants give us energy. They keep us alert. Even the mild stimulants can keep us awake all night. This makes them favorites among truckers hauling overnight loads and students pulling pre-exam all-nighters.

All stimulants decrease our appetite. Mild to moderate stimulants, when used over a period of time, can cause weight loss, thus the market for diet pills. Mild to moderate stimulants can also boost our mental concentration. Methylphenidate helps many people with ADHD to become more focused, in other words, to have an increased capacity for paying attention.

The stronger stimulants pack too much of a wallop to help us pay attention in any sustained sort of way. They get us buzzing with intense sensations of pleasure. They make us feel more like partying than applying our minds to a single task. Like cocaine, the powerful stimulants boost our sense of confidence around others and our feelings of potency within.

Also like cocaine, methamphetamine and methcathinone, when injected, provide a rush. It's blast-off time. Many users describe the rush as a "total body orgasm." In fact, males can experience spontaneous ejaculation during liftoff. Ice, like crack, produces an overwhelming rush of pleasure shortly after the smoke fills the lungs. The rush from ice compares to what we experience from methamphetamine injection.

The Problems They Cause

The problems caused by amphetamines compare nearly identically to those caused by cocaine. (see the subsection "The Problems It Causes" under the "Cocaine" section).

Other stimulants cause the same problems, but the milder the stimulant, the less severe the effect. For example, caffeine causes a rise in blood pressure and heart rate, but to a lesser extent than methamphetamine. And, although overdosing on mild stimulants is rare, some people have done it simply by taking too much on a given occasion.

More on caffeine: I've counseled dozens of clients with severe caffeine addictions, people who down between 12 and 30 caffeine beverages a day. Most of them had been previously addicted to other drugs or alcohol, and this is their "one remaining addiction . . . well, along with nicotine." Most of them had never, or rarely, used harder stimulants. For those who had been addicted to harder stimulants (such as cocaine, amphetamines, or prescription diet pills), excessive use of caffeine would replicate, to some extent, the high they used to experience from the harder stuff. Some of them continue their excessive caffeine use, some have gradually reduced their caffeine consumption to a manageable level, and others have quit the caffeine altogether. Those who don't give up their excessive caffeine consumption relapse more often on the harder stimulants. A couple of years ago, one of my clients overdosed on caffeine and diet pills and spent a week recovering in the hospital. That was her "big crash." After that scare, she quit all stimulants, including caffeine.

Withdrawal

When coming off stimulants, you can expect to feel tired, depressed, and hungry. You might also have little patience, become easily irritated, have a negative outlook on life, or become mentally sluggish. You'll want to sleep, although sleep might not come easily.

When withdrawing from strong stimulants, nothing will seem pleasurable. Things that you would normally enjoy won't be enjoyable, and depression might rule your world.

Most people find that their cravings remain intense for months, even for the mild stimulants. Some people get occasional cravings, even after years of abstinence.

DEPRESSANTS

The depressants include a vast array of synthetic drugs. All but two of them are manufactured as prescription medications by U.S. pharmaceutical companies.

The depressants, also called "downers," have one thing in common. Like alcohol, they depress the central nervous system (CNS), meaning that they reduce the overall nervous activity in the brain and the nervous system. In other words, they calm us. They can reduce anxiety, and they can help us sleep. For this reason, we refer to this whole class of drugs as sedative-hypnotics: "sedative" because of their calming effect and "hypnotic" because they induce sleep. We also know them as "tranquilizers," "anxiolytics," and "anti-anxiety medications."

Options

Chloral hydrate. Synthesized by chemists in the 1800s, this became the first depressant to be widely prescribed, usually as a hypnotic. Over the years, however, its use decreased, especially after the advent of barbiturates in the early 1900s and of benzodiazepines in the 1950s, yet it's still prescribed occasionally today. It has been marketed as a potable syrup and in soft gelatin capsules (trade names: Chloral Hydrate, Notec, Somnos, Felsules). Small doses of this substance, when added to alcohol, will cause an individual to pass out. This led to one of the illegal uses of this drug: spiking someone's drink to knock the person out. Because of this, chloral hydrate acquired the less-than-savory nickname "knockout drops" and, when combined with an alcoholic beverage, became known as a "Mickey Finn."

Barbiturates. The first barbiturate, Barbital, became available as a medicine in the late 1800s. By the 1930s, physicians were prescribing many varieties of barbiturates for numerous complaints. The barbiturates' strong potential for addiction became known by the late 1940s, and by the 1960s pharmaceutical companies began withdrawing products from the market. Besides, these companies began marketing what they called a "safer" and "less addicting" group of depressants known as benzodiazepines. The benzos, it turns out, are just as highly addicting as the barbs, but they do have a much lower potential to cause death by overdose. At one time there were nearly 50 different barbiturates available. Today there are only about 15. The barbs became one of the most widely abused classes of drugs in the 1960s and 1970s. AKA for barbiturates in general: Barbs, Downs, Bears, Goofballs, Fool Pills, Sleeping Pills, Stumblers.

Researchers classify the barbiturates into four categories, depending on the duration of their effects and how quickly their effects begin. The ultra-short-acting produce anesthesia within about one minute after injection. Those in current use (along with trade names) include methohexital (Brevital), thiamylal (Surital), and thiopental (Pentothal). Short-acting and intermediate-acting barbs include pentobarbital (Nembutal), secobarbital (Seconal), amobarbital (Amytal), and a combination of amobarbital and secobarbital (Tuinal). Typically, these have been the preferred barbiturates among barb abusers. Other short-acting to intermediate-acting barbs include butalbital (Axotal, Esgic, Fiorinal, Fioricet), butabarbital (Butisol), talbutal (Lotusate), and aprobarbital (Alurate). The onset of action for these is 15 to 40 minutes, and the effects last up to six hours. Physicians prescribe these for both their sedative and their hypnotic effect. Long-acting barbs include phenobarbital (Luminal) and mephobarbital (Mebaral). The onset of action for these is one hour, and the effects last up to 12 hours. Physicians prescribe these for seizure disorders or the treatment of anxiety. AKA for Amytal: Blues, Blue Devils, Blue Tips, Blue Birds, Blue Heavens, Blue Dolls, Blue Bullets. AKA for Luminal: Purple Hearts. AKA for Nembutal: Nebbies, Nimbies, Yellows, Yellow Jackets, Yellow Dolls, Yellow Bullets. AKA for Seconal: Reds, Red Devils, R.D., Seekies, Red Birds, Mexican Reds.

Barbiturate-like drugs. Pharmaceutical companies developed two depressants, glutethimide and methaqualone, as "similar but safe alternatives" to barbs. However, both proved to be just as addicting as barbiturates, and their potential for overdose was just as great. Even worse, emergency medical personnel find overdoses from these two drugs more difficult to treat than overdoses from barbiturates. Glutethimide (trade name: Doriden) was first available in 1954 and methaqualone (Quaalude, Sopor) in 1965. Because of the frequency of overdose deaths from these two drugs, U.S. pharmaceutical companies stopped manufacturing methaqualone in 1984, and the U.S. Drug Enforcement Agency put tighter controls on glutethimide in 1991. There was some underground production of methaqualone after 1984, but the drug kept losing in popularity and by the mid-1990s was virtually unavailable on the streets. Other barbiturate-like medicines include ethchlorvynol (Placidyl), ethinamate (Valmid), and methyprylon (Noludar). Physicians don't prescribe the barbiturate-like medicines very much anymore. When they do, it's usually as hypnotics. AKA for methaqualone: Ludes, Soapers, Quads, Sopes.

Meprobamate. First marketed in 1965, this drug reduces anxiety and muscle spasms. Also, at therapeutic doses it's not as toxic as the barbiturates or barbiturate-like drugs. It's still occasionally prescribed today. Trade names: Miltown, Equanil.

Benzodiazepines. In 1957, the first benzodiazepine (trade name: Librium) entered the scene. Today, about 15 benzodiazepines are marketed in the United States and another 20 in other countries. They're some of the most widely prescribed drugs in the world, and it's no wonder. This group of sedative-hypnotics does it all. They produce sedation, relieve anxiety, induce sleep, decrease muscle spasms, prevent seizures, and act as an adjunct to anesthesia.

Shorter-acting benzos, used mainly as hypnotics, include estazolam (ProSom), flurazepam (Dalmane), quazepam (Doral), temazepam (Restoril), and triazolam (Halcion). Longer-acting benzos, prescribed mainly as sedatives, include alprazolam (Xanax), chlordiazepoxide (Librium), chlorazepate (Tranxene), diazepam (Valium), halazepam (Paxipam), lorazepam (Ativan), oxazepam (Serax), and prazepam (Centrax). Doctors prescribe clonazepam (Klonopin) mainly for seizure disorders and midazolam (Versed) as an aid to anesthesia. One benzo, Flunitrazepam (Rohypnol), has been gaining popularity as a party drug. It's not marketed in the United States, but it is smuggled in from other countries where it's legal. AKA for Librium: Libs, Libbies. AKA for Valium: V. AKA for Rohypnol: Roofies, Ruffies, Roaches, Trip-And-Fall, Mind Erasers, Mexican Valium.

GHB. Gama-hydroxybutyrate (GHB) is another CNS depressant. It causes intense drowsiness, some-times unconsciousness, and even coma. It can also cause amnesia: the loss of memory for what happened when you were high. This drug is not legally produced in the United States but comes out of clandestine labo-ratories. Like Rohypnol, it has gained recent popularity as a party drug. AKA: GBH, Grievous Bodily Harm, Liquid Ecstasy, Liquid X, Georgia Home Boy, Easy Lay.

Combinations. Many heroin and cocaine users also take depressants—sometimes to augment their buzz on heroin or cocaine and sometimes to ease their tensions when coming down. Some people get ad-dicted to various combinations of ups and downs, often taking ups all day long and downs at night. A combination of Doriden and codeine has become pop-ular with some users (AKA: Dors and Fours).

How They're Used

Almost invariably, people take depressants orally by capsule or tablet or in liquid preparations. The onset of action for the depressants varies from one minute to one hour, and the duration of the high varies from a half-hour to half a day. GHB comes as a white powder that users often mix with water and then drink.

Popularity

SAMHSA's 1996 *National Household Survey on Drug Abuse* divided the depressants into two groups of drugs: "sedatives" and "tranquilizers." The sedatives included all the barbiturates, the barbiturate-like drugs, the hypnotic benzos, and chloral hydrate. The tranquilizers included the remaining benzos and meprobamate. Respondents were not asked about Rohypnol and GHB.

The survey showed that 2.3% of Americans have used illicit sedatives at some time in their lives. About 0.3% have used illicit sedatives in the past year, and 0.1% have done so within the past month. That's about 232,000 current users. The percentages who used illicit tranquilizers were 3.6% lifetime, 1.1% during the past year, and 0.4% during the past month. That's 952,000 current users. (Note: These two categories aren't mutually exclusive. Some people who abused sedatives might have also abused tranquilizers.)

The Joy of It

When we pop a downer, the tension floats away. Our cares float away. Everything is relaxed. Everything's soft—no hard edges here, no raw nerves.

On downers, we get that peaceful, easy feeling. We feel calm inside. Some of us feel smoother in social situations.

When completely downed out, the body seems to disappear while the brain enjoys complete tranquility. In this deep chasm of thought, the body often remains statuesque, acting as if any movement from it would disturb some significant portion of the universe.

The Problems They Cause

Impaired performance. At feel-good doses, the depressants cause slurred speech, dizziness, poor coordination, and poor performance on physical tasks, such as driving a car.

Impaired thinking. When high, users become easily confused and disoriented. They typically experience poor memory, decreased comprehension, faulty judgment, and the inability to focus their attention.

Decreased REM sleep. REM stands for "rapid eye movement." During sleep, REMs occur when we're dreaming. They're a key component of restful sleep. The depressants suppress REMs, creating an interesting dilemma. Although most depressants can be used to help us get to sleep, they diminish the quality of sleep. This causes us to sleep longer than we normally would and to feel sleepy when we awaken.

Nausea. The use of chloral hydrate or GHB causes nausea in most people and vomiting in some.

Seizures. GHB causes epileptic seizures in some users.

Date rape drugs. In recent years, two different drugs (Royhpnol and GHB) have been used in many reported cases of date rape. When combined with alcohol, small doses of either of these drugs can produce physical helplessness, unconsciousness, and amnesia. A perpetrator will drop one of these drugs into an alcoholic beverage that he then hands to a potential victim. After this crime, the perpetrator then commits another: When the victim becomes helpless to resist, he rapes her.

What's happening here? It's one thing to take a chance by putting a drug into your own body. It's quite another thing to sneak a drug into someone else's body. From one viewpoint, it's downright pernicious.

From another, it's immoral and just plain mean. A few of these victims have died. The reason? Alcohol and downers potentiate each other and when combined at even moderate doses can cause death.

(Note: It's illegal to administer a drug to another person without that person's knowledge and with the intent to commit a crime of violence. This is punishable by up to 20 years in prison and a fine.)

Danger of overdose. The potential for overdose runs high for the barbiturates, the barbiturate-like drugs, and chloral hydrate. In overdose, these drugs can produce any or all of the following: respiratory arrest, circulatory collapse (due to extremely low blood pressure), depressed heart function, stupor, coma, and death.

Users of benzos run a lower risk of overdose than users of other depressants. However, the risk of overdose from all the depressants, including benzos, increases dramatically when any of these drugs are combined with each other or with other CNS depressants, such as alcohol, opiates, or inhalants.

Withdrawal

Of all the drugs of abuse, the downers produce the most dangerous withdrawal syndrome. In fact, breaking off a moderate to heavy habit, cold turkey, can kill you. Seizures, high blood pressure, and heart attack can take you away. The more extensive your addiction, the more severe the withdrawal symptoms become. These symptoms include anxiety, agitation, irritability, increased heart rate, panic attacks, hyperactive reflexes, and insomnia. Some symptoms can last up to six months or perhaps even as long as a year.

You can also experience nausea and vomiting as well as confusion, delirium, and hallucinations. These symptoms usually disappear within a few days to a few weeks.

(Note: If you have a moderate to heavy habit, find a physician to manage your withdrawal. Under medical supervision, you'll step down to gradually lower doses over a six- to 12-week period.)

PCP AND KETAMINE

Both PCP (phencyclidine) and ketamine were originally developed by pharmaceutical companies as general anesthetics. However, these drugs also produce mild to severe hallucinations and dissociation—the feeling that you've been separated from your body. For this reason, many researchers refer to PCP and ketamine as "dissociative anesthetics."

Options

PCP. This substance was prescribed for a few years as a general anesthetic under the trade name Sernyl. However, a significant percentage of people, on awakening from PCP anesthesia, experienced excessive agitation, seizures, hallucinations, or delirium. That's why, in 1965, the use of PCP as an anesthetic for humans was discontinued. After that, it was used as a veterinary anesthetic but in 1978 was discontinued for that use as well. Since then, all production of this drug has come out of clandestine labs. AKA: Angel Dust, Peace Pill, Rocket Fuel, Embalming Fluid, Horse Tranquilizer, Elephant Tranquilizer, Monkey Dust, Gorilla Biscuits, D.O.A. (Dead On Arrival).

Ketamine. This PCP congener followed a similar path as PCP. It was first introduced in the United States in 1971 as an anesthetic drug. However, as was found with PCP anesthesia, people awakening from ketamine anesthesia showed signs of delirium and were often hallucinating, although the physical symptoms were not as severe as with PCP. In fact, a benzodiazepine can significantly reverse the side effects of ketamine, and because of this ketamine is still occasionally used in conjunction with a benzo as a human anesthetic. Veterinarians began using ketamine years ago as an anesthetic and still use it to today. The ketamine sold on the streets has most often been diverted from legal markets. AKA: Special K, K, Super C.

Other phencyclidines. By making a change or two in the production phase, illegal manufacturers have created many PCP look-alikes that have similar psychoactive effects. These drugs include PCE, PCPy, TCP, and TCPy. All these have found their way onto the streets, often being sold as PCP, LSD, or some other hallucinogen.

Combinations. Some users smoke marijuana laced with PCP (AKA: Angel Dust, Angel Poke, Supergrass, Wackey Weed, Killer Weed).

How They're Used

The dissociative anesthetics come as pills for swallowing, powders for snorting, rocks for smoking, or solutions for injecting. Dealers have also created smokable combinations by impregnating tobacco, marijuana, parsley, or oregano with one of the dissociative anesthetics.

The high from PCP hits within 15 to 30 minutes and remains at peak levels for four to six hours. However, the drug metabolizes slowly, and because of this significant levels can be found in the body up to two days after taking a single dose. In other words, the high lingers for a couple of days.

The effects from ketamine are not so dramatic. The high comes on within 15 to 45 minutes and lasts four to six hours, but it metabolizes faster than PCP. The high from snorting the powder remains intense for about one hour.

Popularity

About 3.2%, or 6,755,000, of Americans have used PCP at some time in their lives. About 0.2%, or 382,000, have used PCP within the past year. Statistics on the illicit use of ketamine are not yet available.

The Joy of It

Probably more than any other drug, the phency-clidines and ketamine stir excitement through the wild, unpredictable ride. Users hop aboard this un-stoppable though imaginary dreamship that departs from plain, normal, everyday life into the bizarre reaches of lost-in-space psychosis. Most users experience vivid hallucinations. Many users experience racing thoughts as well as "racing bodies"—a physical jacking that makes users want to run around and do things. However, some users get the opposite physical effects. Although their minds fly, their bodies become dead weights, anesthetized as it were and not a matter of present concern. With most users, the mind seems to leave the body, creating a dissociative state that is typical to these drugs.

The Problems They Cause

Physical. These drugs can bring on nausea and possibly vomiting. They commonly cause slurring of speech, muscle rigidity, staggering, grinding of teeth, elevated body temperature, increased heart rate, elevated blood pressure, increased salivation and tearing, and flushing of the skin. These drugs can increase (or decrease) the rate of breathing, depending on the dose.

Mental. Users commonly experience illogical or disorganized thinking, delusions, hallucinations, and an inability to concentrate.

Behavioral. Behavior often becomes unpredictable. Some users become violent. Some get involved in dangerous acts, often while entertaining the delusion that they're impervious or invincible. Some become extremely hyperactive, bouncing off the walls, whereas others become lethargic to the point of catatonia. This is dose related as well.

As noted by drug researchers from the Duke University Medical Center in their book *Buzzed*, "[T]aking PCP can produce a state similar to getting drunk, taking amphetamine, and taking a hallucinogen simultaneously. . . . Many of PCP's bad side effects also resemble those of amphetamine such as increased blood pressure and body temperature. However, at the same time it causes a 'drunken' state characterized by poor coordination, slurred speech, and drowsiness. People under the influence of PCP are also less sensitive to pain. Finally, at higher doses it causes a dissociative state in which people seem very out of touch with their environment. . . . So in total you have someone running around drunk, insensitive to pain, and very uninhibited. Is it any wonder that PCP-intoxicated people find themselves in trouble with the law?"

Psychosis. As with the hallucinogens, PCP and ketamine produce a state resembling psychosis in most users. However, users are less likely to realize that their delusions and hallucinations are just that. In other words, they're more likely to interpret these as real and thus are more likely to make mistakes while high.

In addition, the psychotic state produced by PCP and ketamine takes much longer to go away than that of other hallucinogens. It can last for days from a single dose. As with other hallucinogens, PCP and ketamine sometimes trigger a psychosis that becomes lifelong.

Danger of overdose. Users who "dose up" on PCP or ketamine run the risk of overdose and possibly death. When users double or triple the initial dose or take additional doses before the original high wears off, they begin to experience dangerous side effects. These include general anesthesia, a rise in body temperature to as high as 108 degrees, a rise in blood pressure that can lead to stroke or internal bleeding, muscle damage, kidney failure, liver damage, seizures or epileptic fits, respiratory failure, and coma. Some of these side effects can become so severe that they cause death. The side effects are more severe for the phencyclidines than for ketamine.

Withdrawal

The abstinence syndrome is relatively mild. Coming down from the high usually takes a few days to a week. Then, for an additional week or more, individuals typically feel depressed, and their anxiety level increases. They might also suffer from memory loss.

The emotional depression experienced by short-term heavy users or long-term moderate users can last for months and can even continue for up to a year in recovery. It appears that the pleasure center in the brain needs a long time to recuperate from the dissociative anesthetics.

FOR EXPLORERS

For anyone seeking more information, I recommend the following books:

Buzzed: The Straight Facts About the Most Used and Abused Drugs from Alcohol to Ecstasy, by C. Kuhn, S. Swartzwelder, and W. Wilson. New York: W.W. Norton, 1998.

Drug and Alcohol Abuse: The Authoritative Guide for Parents, Teachers, and Counselors, by H.T. Milhorn. New York: Plenum Press, 1994.

From Chocolate to Morphine: Everything You Need to Know About Mind-Altering Drugs, by A. Weil and W. Rosen. New York: Houghton-Mifflin, 1993.

Street Drugs (revised edition), by A. Tyler. London: Hodder and Stoughton, 1995.

CHAPTER 2

A New View of Drug Addiction

A moment's insight is sometimes worth a life's experience.

—Oliver Wendell Holmes, Sr.

Knowledge is power.

—Francis Bacon

The more you know about a problem, the better equipped you are to resolve it. In this chapter, you'll learn more about drug addiction—why you crave a particular drug and what it gives you in return.

Drug addiction changes everything about you. It becomes a way of life, a deeply ingrained pattern with physical, emotional, and even spiritual edges. There are many parts to it. With the new perspective on drug addiction presented in this chapter, you'll take a look at addiction from the user's point of view. This will help you get acquainted with the user—and the nonuser—inside of you. Then, when you're ready to quit, you can become the nonuser without any fear of drugs.

This seven-part perspective shows how drugs affect the whole person. As you read it, you'll gain a complete understanding of addiction. You'll not only look at the benefits that you gain from a particular drug but you'll also examine the problems it causes.

A WAY OF COPING

Drugs help us cope. Our drug use makes us feel better or helps us avoid some problem. Basically, we use drugs to gain some desired effect. In fact, there are hundreds of ways drugs seem to help, and each person has his or her own unique set of reasons for using them. Here are a few specific ways that drugs help. They can help you:

Take risks

Calm yourself down

Energize yourself

Overcome shyness

Avoid feelings of loneliness

Forget some sadness

Feel bolder

Get into a partying mood

Celebrate happy occasions

Fit into social situations

Feel sexy

Stimulate your desire for sex

Overcome depression

Solve problems

Forget about problems

Stop worrying

Get to sleep

Wake up from sleep

Suppress your anger

Get your anger out

Cope with stress

Reduce feelings of guilt or shame

Ease tensions

Get rid of aches and pains

The ways are countless—for each of us. So much so that often it seems that drugs can cure all our ills and help us overcome whatever bothers us. If that's all there were to it, we might consider each drug to be some kind of "wonder drug." So what's the drawback?

With so many good effects from using drugs, why would anyone want to quit? There are two main reasons: First, if you use excessively, drugs soon stop helping you and actually begin to hurt you. They begin to cause more problems for you than they help you solve. Second, most of us, sooner or later, realize that we would rather do something on our own instead of depending on a drug to help us do it.

Early in our drug-using careers, we're amazed at how easily we can fit drugs into our lives. But it gets harder and harder. Instead of using a drug to help us now and then, we begin depending on it to help us constantly. We feel we can't get along without it. We stop wanting the drug and start needing it.

This is a crucial change. It indicates addiction.

Here's another way to see this change. We start using the drugs to cope with problems that only the drugs are causing. We need a drug to calm us from the effects of getting high the day before, to stop the jitters, or to cut the pain of withdrawal. Sometimes we use one drug to reverse the problems caused by another drug.

Even at this stage, we still have reasons for using. But now the problems from yesterday's drug use become today's reasons for using. That's how powerful a drug of abuse can be. It medicates us from so many problems—even from the problems that it itself causes. No wonder we feel we need it!

It's true that drugs help us cope in many ways. Later, in Chapter 4, you'll list specific ways that drugs help you. Then, in Chapters 5 through 16, you'll discover many different ways of coping—ways that, in the long run, will work better for you than drugs ever did.

SOMETHING YOU LEARN

We don't inherently know how to use drugs. It's something we have to learn. In fact, each drug has its own separate learning curve. The more we use a drug and the more drugs we use, the more there is to learn.

Some of this learning can be fun. When we first start using, we learn the many ways that drugs can help us. We think it's great. Then we begin the long process of learning how to gain the most benefits every time we use. However, that means that we also spend a lot of time learning to minimize the many problems that drugs can cause.

For example, Jeanette learned early on that downers helped her overcome shyness. It helped so much that she quickly began to use them in all social situations. She practiced taking just enough to get the right "buzz" for every occasion. She worked on it long and hard. She had to learn how to take the right amount so she wouldn't get too downed out. She had already learned that whenever she got too downed out, she became completely uncool.

If you use a drug excessively, you have a few main goals. One is learning to create "just the right effect." You have to learn not to overdo it. You attempt to get the perfect buzz. Every time.

But this is difficult. You have to learn your limits. If you take in too much drug at too quick a rate, you might become sick or cause an embarrassing scene. You might get in a bad mood or just get downright sloppy. You might get in trouble with the law, or you might get violent and hurt someone you really care about. Of course, with some drugs, if you do too much too fast, you run the risk of overdose. This can lead to permanent physical or mental damage, coma, or death.

How can you control your drug use all the time? It's hard. In fact, it's damned near impossible. There are just too many variables. For example, each time you get high, that high is different from any other you've ever experienced. Each high varies depending on the following:

1. What your mood was before you started using
2. What drug you're using (including what it was cut with)
3. What other drugs you're using at the same time
4. How long since your previous high on this drug
5. How long since your previous high on some other drug
6. How much you've eaten, what you've eaten, and when
7. How many other toxins your liver is struggling with (e.g., food preservatives and chemical additives, environmental toxins from the air or water, other drugs you've taken, and how much alcohol, nicotine, caffeine, or sugar you've consumed)

8. How you're consuming your drug (swallowing, snorting, sniffing, smoking, or shooting), how fast you're consuming it, and what strength it is

9. Other variables, such as time of month (for women especially, but men also have monthly biological cycles), outside stress factors in your life, or whether your body is fighting a sickness, even if it's something as simple as a sore throat

That's a lot to learn. But as dedicated drug users, we attempt to learn it all. Our purpose? To gain control—so we can get as high as we want, whenever we want, without overdoing it. Some of us become so adept that we can control these variables most of the time.

However, when you get this good, surprisingly there's not much excitement anymore. You normally follow the same routine every day. You maintain a steady habit, and after a while it gets very boring. Most users lose control of their drug intake—not all the time, but often. In some ways it's more exciting to lose control once in a while, but it's also dangerous. When we get too high, accidents can happen—serious accidents. So we try to control the uncontrollable. We try to minimize the danger of hurting ourselves and others. Each time we use, we think, "I can control it if I try." And we keep trying. And trying.

JUST A PART OF YOU

Frank stayed high on marijuana 24 hours a day, seven days a week. He would tell his friends, "I know I'm an addict. There's no two ways about it." Then he would casually fire up another jay.

Actually, there *are* two ways about it. A part of you can be addicted while another part of you can't. In fact, a part of you remains nonaddicted no matter how much you use.

This is very important. Why? Because most people label themselves one thing or another, as addicted or not addicted, but not something in-between. Then they act as if they're stuck in their description and have no choice.

Even if you're a heavy user, even if you stay high constantly, only a part of you can be considered "an addict." Even though all your cells contain traces of your drug, and even though each cell craves that drug as soon as the drug level goes down, each cell still retains some integrity. This integrity is provided by the alternatives to your drug: the food you eat, the water you drink, the air you breathe. To be sure, a definite part of you doesn't depend on that drug. In fact, this part dislikes the drug intensely and fights against it. This part works to preserve your body's natural health.

Rhonda's friends and family members could easily see both sides of her. They would say, "She's okay . . . especially when she's not using the tranquilizers," or, "I know deep down in her heart she's a good person . . . if only she wouldn't take so many pills."

Look inside yourself. Look closely, and you'll see two opposing forces. One of them is an addict. The other is not.

The part of you that's not an addict lies just below the surface, close at hand. But, as you might expect, the higher you are on drugs, the harder it is to get in touch with this part. Still, it's there, and it's very strong. This *non-addicted part* of you has a lot of character. It's an interesting side of yourself that you probably don't know too well. The drugs keep it hidden.

Yet it's this nonaddicted part of you that thinks you might be "addicted." It's there the morning after, shuddering and shaking at what you've done to yourself the night before. The nonaddicted part of you knows that you have a problem.

It's the *addicted part* of you that thinks you're fine. This part keeps excusing the way you act when you're high and keeps hiding your problems from you. This part will do virtually anything to keep you using.

It's the *non-addicted part* that sees the problems that drugs are causing you. This part wants to quit using. This is the part of you that has decided to read this book. It is this part you need to get to know.

Why? Because the nonaddicted part of you will win your battle against drugs. This whole side of you begins to grow as soon as you quit using. Best of all, this side will help you live a longer, healthier, and more fulfilling life than you can ever experience by living through your addicted side.

YOUR OWN SPECIAL STRUGGLE

Some of us might find happiness if we would quit struggling so desperately for it.
—William Feather

Drug use involves you in a struggle—one part of you going one way, one part of you going another. You fight with yourself. And you fight with the drugs to get what you want. The reason? Drugs help you, but they hurt you, too. Your thrills tonight become high blood pressure, headaches, nausea, and regrets tomorrow.

But using is a challenge. And challenges are fun, right? Drugs challenge you to get the benefits they bring while finding ways to avoid the problems. Hey, it's not easy! You try not to get too wiped out here, not to make a fool of yourself there. It's a full-time job. You work hard at it. You juggle your schedule to fit as much of your favorite drug into your life as possible. You find novel ways to handle withdrawals. With some drugs, this becomes a monumental struggle as withdrawals get worse and worse. If you're responsible for making money, you make an extra effort to get to work on time. You try not to get high on the job, or else not to get too high. Sometimes you feel completely helpless. Often you endure a lot of pain.

You would think that, if drugs cause such a struggle, it would be easier to quit. And indeed it would be but for the fact that most of us get completely involved with the struggle itself, so much so that it becomes our own personal life struggle, the inner story of our lives. And of course we grow to like it. Here are some reasons we get attached to the struggle of addiction:

1. It's a challenge.
2. It gives us a sense of involvement.
3. It's like a game—we play hard and try to win.
4. Like the concept of "no pain, no gain," sometimes we need to feel as if we're suffering before we can have a good time.
5. It gives us something to complain about.
6. It requires strength to keep it up—so it shows how *tough* we are.
7. It's like an adventure—every time we use, we don't know where it will lead.

You might like the addictive struggle for any, or for all, of these reasons. Most of us get involved in our struggles for many different reasons, and we might even have different reasons on different days.

"You gotta be tough," Lenny used to say as he passed his favorite mirror containing deftly divided lines of coke. Then he would insist, "Here, blow one of these. It builds character."

He was serious, in a joking sort of way, but it's true. Doing drugs does build character. The "drug-addicted character" deals with a deeper life struggle than most people can handle. It's an intense struggle, requiring a great deal of energy.

You feel this struggle every day. You live hard. You go for all the thrills you can get. And even though you look beat most of the time, and even though you feel exhausted, you continue.

But slowly, over time, you begin to lose it no matter how tough you are. Granted, you might continue fighting on the surface, but the drugs keep hurting you inside. Sometimes it feels as if you're fighting for your very life. And, deep down, this is actually what's happening.

The drugs begin destroying your organs faster than your body can repair them. Your drug use starts a disease process in your body and so you begin to have more and more serious illnesses. In a way, it's as if you're deliberately reminding yourself of death so that the life you feel is a true exhilaration.

This requires strength to keep it up. But ultimately you must surrender. You must surrender by giving your life to drugs, or you must surrender by quitting the drugs.

If you choose to quit, you'll find something else to challenge you, something else to give you a sense of involvement—something to work on or spend your time on or something more interesting to struggle with. This book will help you. Here, you'll discover dozens of exciting, workable alternatives—alternatives that will be more thrilling, bring more rewards, and allow you to be a greater success in your life.

A BODY THAT CRAVES

Psychoactive substances might be a free ticket through life if it weren't for the physical addiction. The physical addiction drags you down. You begin using more but enjoying it less.

What happens? You go from wanting to use to a feeling that you need to use. Deep down, your drug of choice becomes your medicine. It seems to cure everything. The problem is that you begin feeling healthy only when you're using, and you feel sick whenever you stop.

For Joan, quitting pot wasn't easy. Every time she stayed off of it for more than a day, she grew nervous and upset and began getting angry at everyone around her. Like clockwork, every time, by the end of the day, she would say, "I can't stand it anymore! I gotta get high." Her use of marijuana no longer seemed a choice.

Joan could go without pot for about a day. Others can go for three or four days or even a week, before they can't stand it anymore and have to toke up. Some users cannot stay straight for more than a few hours without getting symptoms.

Although this description of physical addiction involves marijuana, the same dynamic holds true for other drugs. However, each class of drugs has its own specific abstinence syndrome. In his book *Drug and Alcohol Abuse,* Dr. Milhorn rated the severity of abstinence syndrome for the various classes of drugs. These ratings, which varied on a scale from 0 to 4, with 4 being the most severe, were as follows:

Depressants: 4

Heroin, opiates, and the analgesics: 3

Cocaine, amphetamines, and other stimulants: 2

Marijuana: 2

Phencyclidines: 2

Inhalants: 1

Hallucinogens: 0

The severity of the abstinence syndrome relates directly to the severity of the physical addiction. Thus, these ratings give us an idea about how severe the physical addiction is for each class of drugs.

How long can you stay off your drug of choice before you begin to feel uncomfortable? Or, more significantly, how long can you stay completely straight—not using any drugs—before you begin to feel uncomfortable? This period of time, between stopping your use and feeling that you need to use again, tells you something about the severity of your addiction: The shorter the period, the more severe the addiction.

Two Signs

There are two signs to the physical addiction. First, you begin needing more and more drug to get the same effects. This is called *increasing tolerance.* Second, you begin to feel as if you can't get along without the drug. You feel more and more pain whenever you try to quit. This sign of addiction is called *withdrawal,* also known as the abstinence syndrome.

"Tolerance" describes how much of a drug your body can handle. As your body adjusts to the drug, your tolerance increases. What two bags of heroin did in the beginning might take five, 10, 20, or even more as tolerance increases. Your body finds its limit.

The second sign of physical addiction appears only when you take the drug away. Your body complains out loud, and your nervous system flashes urgent signals to the mind: "Give me another dose to calm me down" or "Give me another dose to pick me up."

As a rule of thumb, the longer and heavier your drug use, the more problems you'll experience during withdrawal. But also, as we just noted, the abstinence syndrome varies according to the type of substance (or substances) you've been using.

Two Causes

Medical research shows two major causes of physical addiction. First, your cells adapt to the drug and, second, your metabolism becomes more efficient.

Adaptation in the cells. To your cells, the drugs you're using become a way of life. Every time you use a drug, your blood carries it to every cell in your body. Your cells adjust. They grow to expect these doses on schedule.

Your cells learn to cope with various drugs by defending themselves against the drugs' toxic effects. Cell walls harden to retain stability and reduce toxic damage. But as your cells get tough against drugs, gradually more and more can be consumed. Your tolerance increases.

In the long run, however, cell walls break down. At this point, your cells not only lose their ability to keep toxins out but also become unable to retain essential nutrients. Many of them stop functioning altogether or start functioning abnormally. That's when your organs (heart, brain, liver, or lungs), which are nothing more than whole systems of cells, begin to fail.

The problem with metabolism. Metabolism is intimately connected to diet. Your body metabolizes food (breaks it down into its constituent parts) to get vital nutrients to all the cells. To serve this purpose, your body can metabolize many different foods and can learn how to gain nutrients from almost any kind of food you give it.

Metabolism also helps to rid the body of unwanted toxins. The liver is the key organ in this process. The liver "sees" drugs as unwanted toxins and begins producing enzymes that will help eliminate them from the body. It produces a different combination of enzymes for each drug. Moreover, the liver becomes extremely efficient at producing these enzymes. The more it "sees" a particular drug, the more efficiently it produces the enzymes that inactivate that drug.

Thus, a drug that you use often will get eliminated from the body with greater and greater efficiency. It's as if the liver begins to "expect" that drug and has enzymes ready and waiting. This is a key reason that tolerance increases, that is, why it takes greater and greater doses of a drug to get the same original effects.

Yet your personal metabolism works differently from anyone else's. Studies show that each individual has a unique biochemical makeup and that individuals differ greatly from one another in the way they metabolize different foods, drugs, or toxins. To give you an idea how much possible variation there is, researchers have presently identified over 3,000 metabolic substances (called "metabolites") and over 1,100 enzymes. Each individual has different proportions of all 4,100 of these biochemicals. Of the enzymes, only about 30 are responsible for metabolizing all drugs.

Also, the mixture of biochemicals varies for each kind of food you ingest. For example, your body uses different biochemicals to metabolize the different classes of foods: meats, grains, vegetables, beans, fruits, and nuts. As you might have guessed, you need a whole different biochemical preparedness to handle drugs, alcohol, sugars, chemical additives, and toxins.

However, your body adjusts to whatever diet you give it, and the most frequent foods in your diet come to be expected. Biochemical pathways become established the more they are used. Thus, if your body doesn't get an expected food, you actually begin to crave it.

In fact, your body becomes addicted to the foods you give it the most. Your metabolism so completely adjusts to your regular diet that any change from this diet becomes increasingly difficult. Ask anyone who has attempted a major shift in diet.

For example, if you eat meat regularly, your metabolism will take a long time to adjust to a vegetarian diet. Although the same nutrients are available, your body doesn't have the biochemical preparedness. The ability is there. Your body can metabolize vegetarian meals. No problem. But to gain the same efficiency with a new diet can take from one to seven years.

The important thing to remember is this: Metabolism depends on diet. For our purposes, "diet" includes not only the nutritious foods but also the non-nutritious foods, such as sugar and alcohol, as well as other substances, such as chemical additives in foods, environmental toxins, and drugs. You can change your metabolism if you change your diet. Although it will take a long time to change your metabolism significantly, you'll feel incredible improvements after just a few months. You'll discover the kinds of changes you need to make in Chapter 7.

A BRAIN THAT CRAVES

All drugs of abuse have one thing in common: They're fat soluble enough to get into the brain and, once there, to alter its neurochemistry. Most drugs of abuse affect the neurochemicals that activate the brain's pleasure circuits. These drugs reward us with feelings of pleasure.

Only a minority of us become addicted to drugs, but for those who do, it's the feelings of pleasure that become so completely compelling. The brain loves the pleasurable sensations. The brain loves this so much that it gets addicted. That's why the brain begins to crave the pleasure-producing drugs every time we stop using them. This mental attachment to drugs, this craving, has become known as the "psychological addiction."

Some drugs have little effect on the brain's pleasure circuits. For example, the hallucinogens stimulate serotonin, a neurochemical found mainly in the cortex of the brain. This is the site in the brain where abstract thinking occurs. Perhaps because of this, the hallucinogens are less psychologically addicting than drugs such as cocaine or heroin, which stimulate the pleasure center directly.

Also, drugs that stimulate the pleasure center during the "high" cause the reverse effect during withdrawal. During withdrawal nothing seems pleasurable. Life itself becomes raw and painful. Depression sets in. The deeper we get into our addiction, the more extreme each withdrawal becomes and thus the stronger our psychological craving for the drug.

In his booklet *Drugs of Abuse*, Dr. Samuel Irwin rated the psychological addiction potential for various drugs. The ratings, based on a scale from 0 to 5, with 5 being the highest, are as follows:

Heroin: 5

Stimulants (cocaine and amphetamines): 5

Sedatives: 4

Marijuana: 3

Inhalants: 3
PCP: 3
LSD: 2

Avoiding Misery

We become addicted to drugs partly as a way to avoid life's misery. In our minds at least, we become unwilling to suffer.

Real life is loaded with suffering. We not only experience myriad physical pains but also must cope with psychological pain. Many events make us ache inside. Things happen that cause us to feel sad, miserable, angry, nervous, tense, disgusted, confused, weakened, tortured, cheated, abused, frightened, or upset.

But we can avoid these feelings—at least for the moment—by using drugs. We can do drugs and almost instantly feel "high." We can forget about life for a while. We can experience pleasure, excitement, power, courage, thrills, joy, enchantment, and a sense of connection with other people and the world around us.

Of course, in the long run drugs become less and less effective at bringing these benefits. Over time, the drugs themselves start causing suffering. Soon, we find we're using drugs to relieve the misery that drugs themselves have caused. This is known as the "vicious cycle of addiction."

It goes something like this: Life doesn't feel too good. Bang! Try this drug or that drug, and things feel better. Come down off the drug, and things feel worse, just a little worse than they did before you took the drug in the first place. No matter. Bang! Use the drug and feel good again. Gradually, your biochemistry changes. Your brain learns that it doesn't have to keep producing the chemicals that make you feel good.

These chemicals keep appearing without the brain having to do any work. That's why each time you try to get off the drugs, you feel a little worse than the time before. It becomes harder and harder for you to get off the drugs because you feel so bad whenever you try to stop.

And it all started with suffering, with your inability to accept suffering as an intimate part of life. You can break a drug habit anywhere along the way, or never start with drugs at all, simply by accepting life's suffering and facing the suffering head-on.

This doesn't mean that you will live a sad, miserable, and tormented life. There are plenty of ways you can face your suffering and then cope with it. In fact, once you learn these ways and begin using some of them, you'll feel as if your spirit has been renewed.

Of course, it's your choice.

If you choose drugs to cope with life's suffering, you choose a buy-now-pay-later method. It works in the moment, but it just postpones the suffering. And by postponing it, it builds up, so that when you finally do face it, the suffering is immense. The detoxification from drugs might take a week or two, but the long-term withdrawal, the period of time when your biochemistry (and thus your physical and mental health) returns to normal, can take years. Luckily, during this time, you gradually feel a little bit better, day by day.

This book gives you another choice. In it, you'll find more than 100 techniques to help you quit using drugs. There are physical, mental, emotional, and spiritual techniques. Each one of these offers you another way to cope with some aspect of life's suffering. Each one offers you another way to feel good.

Disease, Health, and Addiction

Is drug addiction a disease? There's much confusion.

Sit for a while in a crack house with any crack star and ask if she has a disease. She'll tell you no, even though she might be quick to admit that she's addicted to crack. But ask any recovering cocaine addict in Narcotics Anonymous (NA). She'll tell you that she has a disease and that she has this disease whether or not she's using.

Each of them is partly right. Drug addiction starts a disease process. This process progresses when you're using. It stops when you stop using. And when you stop using, you can heal much of the damage from the disease if you change your diet and lifestyle.

Drug addiction fits the definition of disease. Like other diseases, drug addiction impairs your health by damaging your cells. Like other diseases, it interrupts your body's vital functions, causing specific symptoms. And like other diseases such as cancer, if it's allowed to continue long enough, it can kill you.

But as a disease, it has an ironic twist. The agent causing the disease acts like a medicine that cures the symptoms. Drug-addicted users actually feel healthier when they're using. Pain and sickness seem to disappear. Unfortunately, the sense of health is artificial. When using, you relieve yourself of the symptoms only. Meanwhile, inside your body, the disease process continues.

Drug use wears out your body and actually speeds up the aging process. Your cells live their lives in the fast lane of chemical stimulation and toxic invaders, grabbing a few thrills but choking on the poisons. You begin to feel worn out. You get physically sick more often, or you feel some slight sickness that lingers and is hard to pinpoint.

When cells don't get sufficient nutrients, or if the cells are harmed too often by toxins in the blood, they stop performing important functions. After a while, whole groups of cells begin giving out, and organs begin to fail. Especially susceptible are the brain, heart, liver, pancreas, intestines, kidneys, and stomach.

BECOMING WHOLE AGAIN

Yes, there is a cure for drug addiction.

Your basic goal: to change your metabolism and your brain chemistry for greater health. This means that you need to eliminate drugs, toxins, and some addictive foods from your diet and change some other parts of your diet as well. It also means that you need to find ways to reduce stress, to accept suffering, and to begin enjoying yourself without using drugs.

Then wait.

Why wait? Because once the healing process begins, it takes time to recover. Your body needs time to repair the damage. Your nervous system needs time to repair the damage. It will take a while for your mind to settle. But the best news is that you begin healing right away. In fact, the healthier your new lifestyle, the faster you'll heal. You can heal most of your cells that have been damaged, at least to some degree. But the biggest thing you have going for you is your body's replacement policy.

Your body creates new cells every day—about 300 to 400 million per day! These new cells replace old and dying cells. When you stop using drugs, the new cells your body creates will not be "drug-addicted" cells. They'll never have experienced drugs. These new cells will be healthy, especially if you continue to follow a healthy diet and lifestyle.

Scientists say that every seven years the body replaces every cell (except nerve cells) at least once. That means that the body renews itself and becomes a new conglomeration of cells—a new you—every seven years!

This new you begins every day. If you pay attention, you can feel it.

CHAPTER 3

Do You Have a Problem with Drugs?

Everything free from falsehood is strength.
—May Sarton

Is drug use causing problems for you? It's up to you to find out. In this chapter, you'll do the following:

1. Take a closer look at your drug use.

2. Learn how much you protect your drug use by denying the problems it causes.

3. Take tests to show whether you have a problem with drugs.

I recommend that you start a notebook now. This notebook will be your own private property. You don't have to show it to anyone. Use it to keep track of your life for a while to understand your connection with drugs. Whenever you have the urge to use, write down your mood at the time, how you feel about life, how your body feels, what your immediate surroundings are, and what you want to change by using drugs. As much as possible, note all the information associated with your use of drugs. Then, as you continue to read the self-help methods in this book, you'll discover hundreds of additional ideas to keep you writing.

YOU'RE THE BEST JUDGE

Take a look at yourself. Basically, you know your own condition. Do you feel that you have a problem with drugs? Somewhere deep inside, you know. Look inside and see what you think. Here's your first test:

Test #1:

> ### One Question
>
> Do you sometimes think you have a drug problem?
> ☐ Y   ☐ N

Your intuition is almost always correct. What you answer is probably true. But how can a one-question test tell you anything? It's simple. Most of the time, you deny the problem or hide from it by making excuses. It's only natural to protect something so dear to you, but your defenses break down once in a while.

So, if you *sometimes* think that you have a problem, you almost certainly do.

Imagine yourself the morning after a night of heavy using. Your body feels brittle and weak and your defenses shattered. You're completely nauseated, and you're in pain. This morning you decide not to do any drugs to calm yourself down or to pick yourself up. And, for the moment, you truly feel the misery that drugs are causing you.

This morning, you've had it. You promise yourself you'll stop using drugs for good. However, by the end of the day, your defenses return. You begin to excuse yourself for "one bad night." You "didn't eat enough last night," or you were "really mad at somebody," or else you find some other excuse for using too much. Then you allow yourself to use "just a little tonight." You say, "It's okay *now* . . . I was just having a couple of problems *yesterday*."

You might go through this hundreds of times before you finally recognize the pattern. I know I did.

How can you recognize the pattern of drug addiction, also known as "problem using"? Here's a handy definition to guide you. "Problem using" means that you're using *too much, too often,* and that you're *out of control.* Let's look at this three-part definition.

Once again, trust your own judgment. If you feel you're using too much on certain occasions, your feeling is probably correct. If you feel you're getting high too often, your feeling is probably correct. If you feel it's happening because you can't control it, you're probably addicted. If drugs eliminate your self-control, or if getting high alters your personality, you almost certainly have a problem.

Pay attention to your deepest feelings. Try writing them in your notebook. Write how you feel about your drug use, how you feel about how much and how often you use, and what kind of control you have over it. You don't need to analyze it. Just say what you feel—it might surprise you.

STOP HIDING

He who conceals his disease cannot expect to be cured.

—*Ethiopian proverb*

Heavy users like getting high so much that they'll do almost anything to protect their habits. Do you protect your drug habit? When drugs cause problems, do you try to deny the problems or minimize them? There are three main ways you might be protecting your drug use:

1. You might deny how serious the problems are.

2. You might deny that drugs cause the problems.

3. You might make excuses for using.

Heavy users incorporate all three ways to hide from their problems. You'll find a list of specific denials and excuses that people use in Worksheet #1 at the end of this section.

Each user has an elaborate system of denials and excuses. Bill denied his problems with cocaine and amphetamines and made excuses to suit his needs. In fact, he enjoyed the challenge of it. Whenever anyone suggested that he had a problem with his use of drugs, he had another excuse. It was like playing a game of chess—and he was very good at staying one move ahead of his opponent. However, this kept him from the truth for a long time—almost too long. When he finally got a medical checkup, he found that his physical problems (with his lungs, liver, and gastrointestinal system) were extremely serious, much worse than he ever admitted to anyone (including himself).

The denials and excuses you make to others are alarming enough, but they become even worse when you start believing them yourself. When this happens, it means that you can maintain a false image of your health for a long time. Meanwhile, problems inside you can be raging out of control and getting worse. Problems all around you—with family, romantic relationships, and friendships—can become more extreme as well. That's why it's important to break this pattern as soon as you can.

How do you break the pattern? One way is to wait until you get a big scare, a near-death experience caused by your use of drugs—something so obvious that you simply can't deny it. It can be a severe health crisis, an accident, or something you did while high that you regret very much. A big scare dissolves all lies. Almost instantly you can see directly into your own reality.

However, if you do have a problem with drugs, this is not the best way to find out. Don't wait to get a jolt like this because you might not survive it.

The other way to break the pattern—the best way—is to simply stop the lies. Then you can see the real you and the real problems that drugs are causing. Once you can detect the lies, you can stop them. The following worksheet will help you.

Worksheet #1

Denials and Excuses

Instructions. Look over the following lists and check the denials and excuses you use. Return to this worksheet periodically, maybe every 2 weeks for a couple of months, to make sure you don't miss anything. Add your own excuses if you don't find them listed here. Also, write the exact wording whenever you can. When you know the exact words you use, you can see more clearly what you're trying to hide. Go over your list now and then, until you feel it's complete. (Work here, on these pages, or work in your notebook.)

Denials I Use

Denying the Seriousness of Problems

- ☐ I'm not addicted. I can stop whenever I want.
- ☐ I don't have any problems with drugs. My drug use isn't a problem.

☐ I'm using drugs for a good purpose. It helps me with

_____.

☐ Drugs are like a medicine to me.

☐ I don't use too much. Just a few hits/snorts/sips/shots/ pills now and then. (Check here if you use this lie to convince others that you don't use too much. Check here also if you hide your drug use from family members or friends.)

☐ Sure I might use a lot, but drugs never get the best of me.

☐ I can always make it to work on time; or, I can always get the meals cooked and the clothes washed (or anything that suggests you meet your responsibilities in spite of your drug use).

☐ (Referring to any kind of internal problem): It's just a little pain. It usually goes away when I get high.

☐ Well, I made it home all right, so everything must be okay; or, I didn't get picked up by the police, so I must have driven okay. (Then you look at your car and see a scrape): Well, it's only a scrape. There's no blood, so it's okay.

☐ It was an accident. Accidents happen to everybody.

☐ It's just a minor problem. It doesn't do too much harm.

Other ways you deny the seriousness of drug-related problems:

☐ _____
☐ _____
☐ _____
☐ _____
☐ _____
☐ _____
☐ _____

Denying That Drugs Cause the Problems

☐ I was nervous as hell. I simply had to have a hit/snort/ sip/shot/pill (instead of realizing that your nervous tension was caused by withdrawal from drugs).

☐ I was feeling so down that I needed a pick-me-up (denying that your feelings were caused by drug withdrawal).

☐ I was really upset, so I used just a little (once again, denying a sign of withdrawal).

☐ It's not the drugs that make me this way. It's just me. It's the way I am.

☐ It's not the drugs that are messing me up. My life's a little crazy, that's all.

☐ It's not the drugs. I've never gotten ahead in life because I don't come from a privileged background.

☐ I didn't lose the job because of my drug use. The boss was just out to get me; or, That job wasn't "my style," and besides, I never liked it anyway.

☐ These troubles have just started happening lately. I don't know where they come from.

☐ It's not my drug use—it's something else. I just haven't been eating well lately; or, I'm under a lot of pressure lately; or, _____.

☐ Stay out of my business. It's my life, and you don't know anything about what's wrong with me (whenever someone suggests that you have a problem with drugs).

☐ It's not the drugs. It's the cigarettes; or, It's the coffee; or, it's that damned alcohol.

☐ I must be constipated (or, I must have diarrhea) because of the food I ate, not because of the drugs.

☐ Gee, this pain in my right side (liver) is really bothering me. I wonder what's wrong. (You can use this same kind of denial with many physical symptoms, pretending that drugs have nothing to do with the symptoms):

    ☐ This pain in the middle of my back (kidneys)

    ☐ This pain in my left side (pancreas)

    ☐ My high blood pressure

    ☐ That damned ulcer

    ☐ My unclear thinking

    ☐ _____ (See Worksheet #3 in Chapter 4 for other problems that drugs cause that you might be denying.)

Other ways in which you deny that drugs cause problems:

☐ _____

☐ _____

☐ _____

☐ _____

☐ _____

☐ _____

☐ _____

☐ _____

Excuses I Use

Excuses to Start Using

☐ I need a hit/snort/sip/shot/pill to unwind.

☐ I'm having a rough day. I think I'll get high.

☐ Whenever my _____ (wife/husband/girlfriend/
boyfriend/boss/friend/son/daughter/mother/father)
gets mad at me, I just want to get high.

☐ It's attitude-adjustment hour—time to get high!

☐ I had a bad day.

☐ I had a good day.

☐ The sun is shining.

☐ It's cloudy and miserable.

☐ It's cold out! I need a hit/snort/sip/shot/pill to warm
me up.

☐ It's hot outside! I need a hit/snort/sip/shot/pill to cool
me down.

☐ I worked hard and got a lot done. Now I'll reward myself.

☐ I need an eye-opener.

☐ I need a hit/snort/sip/shot/pill to give me a lift.

☐ It helps me put up with some unbearable situation:
_____.

☐ I need a hit/snort/sip/shot/pill to help me
_____. (Fill in the blank with

your reasons for using. See Worksheet #2 for help.
Your reasons for using can quickly become excuses
for using.)

Other excuses you make to start using:

☐ _____

☐ _____

☐ _____

☐ _____

☐ _____

☐ _____

☐ _____

☐ _____

Excuses to Continue Using

☐ I need just one more hit/snort/sip/shot/pill to settle
me down.

☐ Well, I'm started now.

☐ You only live once, so you might as well go for all the
thrills you can get!

☐ Well, if you're offering it for free.

☐ I need another hit/snort/sip/shot/pill to keep me going.

☐ What the hell. Sure, I'll do some more.

☐ I need more to really have a good time.

☐ I need to do more to face _____(a certain
person) or be with _____(a certain
person).

☐ I need more to get in the mood, to get just the right
buzz, just the right glow.

☐ If I have more I'll get rid of this anger (Or any other
bad emotion): _____.

☐ One more for the road.

☐ One more to good friends.

☐ All right, if you insist.

☐ Well, just one more.

☐ One more to help me sleep.

Other excuses you make that keep you using once you start:

☐ _____

☐ _____

☐ _____

☐ _____

☐ _____

☐ _____

☐ _____

☐ _____

Excuses for Using Too Much

☐ I guess I did a little too much last night.

☐ It's not my fault. They kept giving me more. What was I to do?

☐ I shouldn't have been using on an empty stomach.

☐ I got too out-of-it because I was mixing my drugs.

☐ I got too out-of-it because I was shooting instead of snorting.

☐ I couldn't help it. It's just one of those things. I simply had too much, and that's that.

☐ The drugs aren't the problem. I used too much because of my real problem: _____.

☐ I was under too much stress, and the _____ (cocaine, marijuana, whatever drug you were using) helped me feel better.

☐ Sorry, I won't get that way again.

☐ I just forgot to watch how much I was using.

☐ Damn it all! I'll never get that messed up again.

☐ After last night, I never want to touch the stuff. I'm going to quit it for good.

☐ What the hell. I just used too much. It's not the end of the world.

☐ It was an overdose. It wasn't so bad. Anyway, this was just my first one. (Some people will use this excuse for every overdose: "Anyway, this was just my fourth one.")

☐ _____ (name) was worse off than I was.

☐ This time I finally learned my lesson.

☐ Don't worry, it'll pass.

☐ It wasn't my fault. I was just too high to know what I was doing. (Excuses like this get more serious. Instead of excusing your drug use, you excuse bad behavior because of your drug use. For example, after beating your spouse or your child, you say, "It wasn't my fault. I was just too high to know what I was doing.")

☐ Wow! I really got wasted last night, but what a night!

☐ It'll make a good story, won't it?

☐ I forget everything. It's a complete blank.

☐ I'm sorry if I said anything to offend you.

☐ I'm sorry I hit you. The drugs made me do it.

☐ I hope I didn't make any enemies last night or hurt anybody. No, I couldn't have, could I?

☐ If I just apologize for being too messed up, everything will be okay.

Other excuses you make for using too much:

☐ _____

☐ _____

☐ _____

☐ _____

☐ _____

☐ _____

☐ _____

☐ _____

NOW TAKE ANOTHER LOOK

Nothing can be loved or hated unless it is first known.

—*Leonardo da Vinci*

A number of recent Mayo Clinic studies have shown that "paper-and-pencil" tests identify alcohol addiction more consistently and more accurately than laboratory tests. It seems that laboratory tests aren't sensitive enough to catch all the cases. Those who had passed their lab tests but showed signs of alcoholism on their written tests were checked again. Almost invariably, the written test proved correct.

Test #2 can show whether you have a problem with drugs. You'll also learn a little about how bad the problem really is. Give it a try.

Test #2:

Do You Have a Problem with Drugs?

Instructions. Answer the following questions honestly. Then score yourself according to the key. Work here or in your notebook.

1. Have you ever felt you should cut down
   on your drug use?   ☐ Y   ☐ N

2. Do you ever use drugs when you're alone?   ☐ Y   ☐ N

3. Have you ever used more of a drug than
   you intended in a given period of time?   ☐ Y   ☐ N

4. Have you ever used drugs for a longer
   period of time than you originally
   intended?   ☐ Y   ☐ N

5. Have you ever used more than one drug
   at a time?   ☐ Y   ☐ N

6. Concerning your use of drugs, has anyone
   ever told you that you use too much?   ☐ Y   ☐ N

7. Have you ever taken one drug to overcome
   the effects of another?   ☐ Y   ☐ N

8. Have you ever thought that your life
   might be better if you didn't take drugs?   ☐ Y   ☐ N

9. Have you ever felt angry at yourself or guilty because of your drug use? ☐ Y ☐ N

10. Do you regularly use a drug at certain times of the day or on certain occasions, for example, when you go to bed, when you wake up, before or after a meal, or before or after sex? ☐ Y ☐ N

11. Have you ever lied about your drug use to family members or friends? ☐ Y ☐ N

12. Have you ever lied to a doctor or faked symptoms to get prescription drugs? ☐ Y ☐ N

13. Have you ever stolen drugs? ☐ Y ☐ N

14. Have you ever stolen money or material goods that you could sell to obtain drugs? ☐ Y ☐ N

15. Have you ever done things to obtain drugs that you later regretted? ☐ Y ☐ N

16. Has your drug use ever caused problems for you with school or with work? ☐ Y ☐ N

17. Have you noticed that you need to use more and more of a drug to get you high? ☐ Y ☐ N

18. Do you experience withdrawal symptoms when you go without drugs for a few days? ☐ Y ☐ N

19. Do you panic when your drug supply gets low? ☐ Y ☐ N

20. Have you ever done something when you were high that you felt guilty about later? ☐ Y ☐ N

21. Have you ever gotten into fights when high on drugs? ☐ Y ☐ N

22. Have you ever been arrested for any drug-related activity (including possession)? ☐ Y ☐ N

23. Have you ever been diagnosed with a medical problem related to your drug use? ☐ Y ☐ N

24. Have you ever overdosed on a drug? ☐ Y ☐ N

25. Have you ever attended a treatment program specifically related to drug use? ☐ Y ☐ N

26. Have you associated with people with whom you normally wouldn't just so you could have access to drugs?   ☐ Y   ☐ N

27. Have you stopped associating with any of your friends because they don't use drugs as much as you?   ☐ Y   ☐ N

If you answered Yes to any two of these questions, this is a sign that you have a problem with drugs. If you answered Yes to any three, the chances are that you do have a problem with drugs. If you answered Yes to four or more, you definitely have a problem with drugs.

You might want to try more than one test. Here are three other options:

"DSM-IV Substance Abuse Test," in *The Addiction Workbook*, by P. Fanning and J.T. O'Neill. Oakland, CA: New Harbinger Publications, 1996.

"Self-Diagnosis: Critical Questions to Ponder," in *The Recovery Book*, by A.J. Mooney, A. Eisenberg, and H. Eisenberg. New York: Workman, 1992.

"Am I Addicted?" published by Narcotics Anonymous (IP No. 7), P.O. Box 9999, Van Nuys, CA 91409 (Phone: 818-773-9999).

WHAT'S THE VERDICT?

To understand is to forgive, even oneself.
—Alexander Chase

Now that you've taken a closer look, you should know more about your relationship with drugs. What did you learn? After carefully considering your relationship to drugs, did you decide to change anything? If so, what?

As your next step, in Chapter 4 you'll discover more about drug-related problems—and which ones affect you the most. You'll also judge for yourself how serious your problems have become.

If you have a problem with drugs, remember this: You can solve it. You'll soon learn plenty of ways to help yourself. If you've decided that you need to quit drugs right away, complete Checklist #1 in Chapter 4 and read the section just after that to determine whether you need in-patient care for detoxification. Then quit. You can just as easily do the remaining techniques in Chapters 4 through 9 after you quit.

CHAPTER 4

Are the Benefits Worth the Problems?

He who hesitates is sometimes saved.
—James Thurber

Take a moment to consider: How bad is your problem with drugs? How many things have gone wrong in your life since you first started using?

You might have some trouble answering these two questions. Why? Because you keep remembering the benefits you get from using. Drugs help you cope in so many ways that you tend to overlook the problems they cause. You might deny the problems, or you might not realize that drugs are causing many of your problems.

Actually, drugs have many side effects. When you use too much, every living cell in your body is harmed. Over a short period of time, the damage becomes serious. Your vital organs weaken: your brain especially, but also your heart, liver, digestive organs, and sex organs. Because of this, you tend to have thought disorders, heart disease, skin problems, digestive problems, weak bones, sexual dysfunction (including problems with childbirth), nervous disorders, and emotional problems. Furthermore, as your cells become weaker, you become more susceptible to degenerative diseases, such as cancer and AIDS.

In this chapter, you'll weigh the benefits of drugs against the problems they cause and then decide whether you need to quit using. Even if you've already decided to quit, these exercises will help you confirm and strengthen your reasons for quitting.

Back in the early days of Twelve Step programs, it was said that alcoholics and drug addicts had to hit "rock bottom" before they could begin to change. However, this isn't so. With early self-assessment (from the checklists and worksheets in this chapter), you can decide to make a change before you hit rock bottom and in turn save yourself a lot of trouble. Things might be bad now, but you can decide to change before they get worse.

As your first step, take a look at the many different ways in which you use drugs to help you cope.

THE BENEFITS OF USING

Drugs might be hurting you, but you keep using them because they also do something good for you. You use a particular drug to gain certain benefits in life. Ask anyone who has a moderate to heavy habit, and he or she can give you plenty of good reasons for using.

What are your reasons? Complete Worksheet #2 to find out.

Worksheet #2

My Reasons for Using Drugs

Instructions. First, consider all the drugs you use. You might use only one drug, or you might use more than one, but each time you use a drug, you have a reason. What are your reasons? Put a check next to each one of your reasons for using. Check as many reasons as you feel relate to you. Use the blank lines in each category to write any additional reasons you have.

To forget about myself or my problems:

☐ It helps me relax or wind down.

☐ It helps reduce tension.

☐ It helps me stop worrying.

☐ It helps when I'm depressed.

☐ It helps when I feel lonely.

☐ It helps me forget my problems.

☐ It helps me feel better when my life seems hopeless.

☐ It helps when I feel no one cares about me.

☐ It helps me forget painful memories.

☐ Sometimes I use when I feel guilty or ashamed (even when it's my using that I feel guilty or ashamed about).

☐ It helps me forget a serious crisis in my life, such as losing a loved one, a bad accident I had, getting fired. (Write it here): _____

_____

For pleasure, kicks, or the thrill of it:

☐ When I use, I feel I have more fun.

☐ When I'm high, everything I do seems more pleasurable.

☐ The high feels so good, I just want to keep it going.

☐ I use because I love the rush.

☐ Sex feels better when I'm high.

- ☐ Sometimes I get high as a way to celebrate. (It can be anything: a holiday, good news, or a reunion with an old friend.)
- ☐ Sometimes I use for sentimental reasons—to remember something pleasurable in the past.
- ☐ I use because I like the taste of the smoke in my throat and lungs.
- ☐ I like the effects of getting high. I like the sensation it gives me.
- ☐ I like the glow.
- ☐ I do it just for kicks.

To enhance experiences or to explore consciousness:

- ☐ I like the sensory stimulation. (Things look better, sound better, taste better, smell better, or feel better to the touch.)
- ☐ I like using because it gives me a different view of reality.
- ☐ I like the hallucinations.
- ☐ I use because it helps me explore my mind.
- ☐ I like the mental adventure. I like not knowing what to expect next.
- ☐ It helps me think profound thoughts.
- ☐ It makes the world appear more beautiful (or more wondrous).

- ☐ _____
- ☐ _____

To reduce inhibitions, make me feel more powerful, or help me get along with others:

- ☐ When high, I don't feel so shy.
- ☐ It helps me get along in social situations.
- ☐ I feel I perform better sexually.
- ☐ It helps me express my anger.
- ☐ Sometimes I use just to show people I can (especially if they've been telling me they think I should quit).
- ☐ It shows how tough I am. You gotta be tough to use as much as I can.
- ☐ My friends all use, and they expect me to use.

- ☐ It helps me fit in.
- ☐ It makes me feel more mature.
- ☐ It helps me speak my mind.
- ☐ It builds my courage.
- ☐ It helps me face responsibilities.
- ☐ It helps me take risks.
- ☐ It helps me solve problems.
- ☐ It helps me make decisions.
- ☐ It helps me accept failure when things don't work out.
- ☐ When using, I feel more complete, more fulfilled.
- ☐ When I use, I feel more loving.
- ☐ When I use, I feel more independent.
- ☐ _____
- ☐ _____

To sedate me:
- ☐ When high, I don't feel so nervous.
- ☐ It helps me sleep.
- ☐ It helps stop the shakes in the morning.
- ☐ It helps me get rid of pain (headache, muscle pain, toothache, cramps, or any other body ache or pain).
- ☐ It stops me from thinking too much.
- ☐ It helps when I'm feeling stressed.
- ☐ It slows me down when things seem to be going too fast.
- ☐ _____
- ☐ _____

To stimulate me:
- ☐ It picks me up when I'm feeling down.
- ☐ It rouses me when I feel bored.
- ☐ It helps me wake up in the morning.
- ☐ Sometimes I use to stop myself from being hungry.
- ☐ Sometimes I use to make myself hungry.
- ☐ It helps to clear my head.
- ☐ It helps me be more creative (or artistic).

☐ It helps me to perform better (at music, drama, sports, or any other task, such as assembly-line work, housework, home-repair jobs, driving, or studying).

☐ _____

☐ _____

It's automatic, part of my lifestyle:

☐ I have certain times of the day when I use. (For example, in the morning, at lunchtime, after 4:00 PM, just after dinner, or just before bedtime.)

☐ It's the only way I know. It's my lifestyle.

☐ It's automatic. Sometimes I start using without even realizing it.

☐ It's part of my life. I'm attached to it. I'd be completely lost without it.

☐ _____

☐ _____

To satisfy my addiction, to avoid unpleasant feelings of withdrawal:

☐ I can go only a certain amount of time before I need another hit/snort/sip/shot/pill.

☐ Often I feel as if I just have to have the _____ (marijuana, cocaine, Valium, heroin, or whatever your drug of choice).

☐ When I stop using, I start feeling sick.

☐ I use because I don't have a choice. I'm seriously addicted to _____ (drug of choice).

☐ When I use, it kills this irresistible urge—this craving I feel deep inside my gut.

☐ My using stops the cold, clammy feeling I sometimes get when the high starts wearing off.

☐ When I use, it stops the trembling (or the spasms or seizures).

☐ When I use, it stops the mental confusion that happens whenever I come down.

☐ _____

☐ _____

Now take a second look. Maybe you said that using helps calm you down. Maybe that's because your favorite drug acts as a sedative. However, whenever this drug leaves your system, you become more agitated than before you took it. Over time, you need more and more of this drug to calm you down because withdrawal from it makes you more and more agitated. Now, you have to stay high all the time or use a really high dose before you finally feel calm.

Maybe you said that you use drugs to help you have fun. Now, when you use, you don't really have fun. You have memories of fun. Maybe your using has become so serious that it's simply not fun anymore.

Maybe you said that a particular drug helps you have better sex. But now, that same drug often kills your desire or impairs your ability to have sex.

After a while, drugs stop helping you with specific problems, or else you need more and more to overcome these problems. In fact, you might find that drugs don't help you at all anymore, but you continue to use because you remember how they helped you in the past. Many of us keep using for years in an attempt to re-create "the good days." But those days never return.

Now go back over your list and put *a second check* next to anything that drugs *still* help you do. Think about each benefit, and be honest with yourself. Ask, "Does the drug still help me do this?" Undoubtedly, you feel that drugs do still help you in certain ways. Some of the items on your list probably have two checks. However, to quit drugs successfully, you need to find other ways to do what drugs do for you now. The remaining chapters offer you successful methods to gain the benefits you get from drugs without having to use them.

PROBLEMS CAUSED BY USING

How can you know the true value of drugs in your life? You just looked at some of the benefits. Now compare these benefits with some of the problems that drugs cause.

Originally, you started using to gain something—you got certain benefits. However, soon you started using to escape from problems or to forget about how bad you feel. Unfortunately, using too much or too often makes your problems even worse, and it becomes a vicious cycle, a self-defeating mechanism. The very way in which you choose to solve your problems actually aggravates and intensifies them.

What's worse, your drug use causes its own problems—problems that become so serious that they can kill you. You can be assured that heavy drug use will kill you, sooner or later. It's slow suicide for some and fast suicide for others.

Jenna, a speed freak who had been in recovery for more than a year, told me, "It was like being married to someone you love very much, then finding out that person is a beast who's trying to kill you."

At some point you'll discover that your drug of choice is a beast that's trying to kill you—and at that moment your love affair will end.

For the time being, though, you keep the benefits of using in your mind. You *know* them. You *think* about them often. You can put them into words. However, the problems caused by your drug use remain in the body, just under the surface. They're not so obvious, and, chances are, you haven't put them into words. You don't usually think about them or talk about them. Even so, you can find these problems if you take a look. In the next section, you'll take a look.

Are Drugs Hurting You More Than You Know?

Most people know that too much of a particular drug harms their bodies, but how much harm does it do? Practice #1 will help you break through your denials and look at a drug's potential threat to your physical health.

Your body holds many secrets. As drugs compromise your health, your body sends warning signs. Unfortunately, too many users make the mistake of ignoring these important signs.

So here's your chance to unlock these inner secrets. Just take some time and listen to your body. You'll find this exercise works best when you're not using. It can be especially effective the day after a period of heavy use.

Practice #1

Dialogue with the Body

Instructions. Close your eyes and relax. Get as comfortable as you possibly can.

Now go inside yourself and practice centering your attention on different parts of your body. By projecting your mind into your body, you can determine how it feels. Ask your body to tell you how it responds to your drug of choice. Let your mind focus on different organs, glands, and muscles, and, as you do, be sensitive to their condition. Ask each bodily part, "How do you feel about _____ (drug of choice)? How does the drug affect you?" Ask:

    Your feet
    Your legs
    Your back
    Your chest
    Your hands
    Your arms

Your face
Your head

Try touching these areas with your hand as you center your mind on them.

Then allow different organs and organ groups to tell you how they feel about the drug:

Your heart
Your liver (right side at bottom of rib cage)
Your pancreas (left side at bottom of rib cage)
Your throat
Your stomach
Your intestines
Your kidneys (middle of back, both sides)
Your sex organs (organs of reproduction)
Your lungs
Your brain

Again, it helps to touch these areas with your hands as you think about them.

Finally, ask your five senses how they feel about the drug:

Your eyesight (you may open your eyes a few times for this one)
Your hearing
Your sense of touch
Your sense of smell
Your sense of taste

Take as much time as possible with each area of your body. Listen as long as you can before moving on. This might not be easy at first, but be patient. Your body will soon open up to you. If you use more than one drug, try this exercise for each drug you use.

Write your responses in your notebook or use a separate sheet of paper. I suggest putting your comments in writing because it will help you remember them.

I started doing Practice #1 about a year before I had quit smoking pot. What a discovery! I learned how much my body really hated the marijuana. It had been causing anxiety and paranoia for years, serious lung pain, and other physical aches and pains. My body wanted to quit smoking it. Later, when I finally did quit, it helped me to know that some major part of me desperately wanted to make a change.

My body knew the problems that pot was causing. It was my mind that loved it. It was my mind that compelled me to get high. My mind had simply been ignoring my body all those years.

The part of you that's addicted lives in the mind. Your body can be ailing and weeping, yet your mind can still want to use. When you quit your drug use, it helps to get in touch with your body. It helps to get your mind listening to your body more often.

Drugs and Your Health

In this section, you'll discover some specific medical problems that drugs cause. You can discern many of these problems by yourself, but you should plan on getting a physical checkup. This will let you know for sure whether you have a medical condition and how serious it is.

As your first step, you need to find the right doctor. You want a doctor who knows addictions, especially drug addiction. So ask around. Often the best place to go is a clinic specializing in treating drug and alcohol addiction. You don't have to admit yourself for treatment; tell them you just want a medical assessment.

Then plan to tell the doctor everything. First, state that you're concerned about your drug use. Describe as much about your history of using as the doctor wants to know. Be as accurate as possible. In addition, report how you scored on the tests in Chapter 2.

Checklist #1 gives you a fairly complete list of signs, disorders, and diseases common to users of psychoactive drugs. As a user, you run a greater risk than normal of getting any one of these problems. If you have any of them already, it might indicate serious trouble. Even simple visible signs often indicate a deeper problem. For example, red skin blemishes are associated with liver malfunction.

Checklist #1

Medical Problems

Instructions. Follow these three steps:

1. Look over the following "Symptoms" checklist. Put a check next to any symptom that you have now or that you have had in the past 5 years.

2. Share the list with a doctor. These symptoms are signs of deeper problems, so be sure to get tested to determine what deeper problems you might have.

3. What problems did the doctor diagnose? Look over the "Medical Problems" checklist which lists problems common among drug users. Check the problems that have been diagnosed in you.

Symptoms

Liver/Gall Bladder

- ☐ Sensitivity in right abdomen (push two or three fingers into right abdomen, just below ribs)
- ☐ Pains in right abdomen
- ☐ Hardened, enlarged area in right abdomen
- ☐ Swelling of abdomen with fluid (ascites)

☐ Yellowing of skin, yellowing in the whites of eyes, or a
   tan on a light-skinned person even without sun (jaundice)
☐ Vomiting blood

Pancreas/Spleen

☐ Sensitivity in left abdomen just below ribs
☐ Pains in left abdomen

Gastrointestinal

☐ Frequent sore throat
☐ Stomach pain
☐ Stomach cramps
☐ Abdominal pain with meals
☐ Frequent heartburn
☐ Digestive problems
☐ Frequent vomiting
☐ Bowel problems: diarrhea, constipation, or diarrhea al-
   ternating with constipation
☐ Bloody or black stools

Kidneys and Bladder

☐ Pains on either side of the middle of back
☐ Cramps in the middle of the back
☐ Excessive urination (more than ten times a day)
☐ Difficulty or pain urinating
☐ Blood in urine

Nose and Throat

☐ Soreness in the lining of the nose
☐ Nasal bleeding
☐ Hoarseness
☐ Difficulty swallowing

Metabolism

- ☐ Excessive hunger
- ☐ Excessive thirst
- ☐ Frequent headaches
- ☐ Craving sweets
- ☐ Shakiness or nervous tension, especially just before eating
- ☐ Feeling weak
- ☐ Cold, clammy feeling
- ☐ Feeling jittery
- ☐ Confused thinking

Lungs

- ☐ Excessive congestion
- ☐ Difficulty breathing
- ☐ Constant hacking cough
- ☐ Frequent colds
- ☐ Lung pain

Heart and Circulatory System (Cardiovascular)

- ☐ Chest pains
- ☐ Swelling in feet
- ☐ Feet cold and painful
- ☐ Sores that don't heal or heal very slowly
- ☐ Rapid heartbeat (tachycardia)
- ☐ Rapid, irregular heartbeat (palpitations)
- ☐ Abnormal changes in heartbeat (arrhythmia)

Blood

- ☐ Extreme physical weakness
- ☐ Feeling faint
- ☐ Occasional fainting

Joints, Muscles, and Bones

- ☐ Sore joints
- ☐ Sharp pain in joints
- ☐ Frequent broken bones
- ☐ Muscle cramps
- ☐ Muscle pains
- ☐ Poor muscle development or tone

Eyes

- ☐ Dimness of vision, especially night vision
- ☐ Poor vision or problems with vision
- ☐ Repeated eye infections

Sex Organs

- ☐ Decrease in size of testicles
- ☐ Increased vaginal infections
- ☐ Decreased sex drive (male or female)
- ☐ Decreased enjoyment of sex
- ☐ Pain in sex organs
- ☐ Pain during sex

Skin

- ☐ General redness or flushing of skin
- ☐ Rashes
- ☐ Small red blemishes in spider-like pattern (blemishes turn white with pressure)
- ☐ Increase of visible red blood vessels on face
- ☐ Red acne-type skin (rosacea)
- ☐ Dark-red blotches on skin
- ☐ Poor skin condition in general
- ☐ Ulcers of the skin

Other General Signs

- ☐ Poor hair condition
- ☐ Loss of hair
- ☐ Abnormalities in gait
- ☐ Decreased ankle and knee reflexes
- ☐ Increased gag reflex (back of tongue at esophagus)
- ☐ Bleeding gums
- ☐ Sores on the body
- ☐ Bags or circles under eyes
- ☐ Steady weight loss or steady weight gain
- ☐ Overdevelopment of mammary glands in males
- ☐ Frequent accidents

Nervous and Mental Disorders

- ☐ Feeling on edge, jumpy
- ☐ Nervous tension (anxiety)
- ☐ Feeling sad or depressed
- ☐ Shooting pains in extremities
- ☐ Tingling sensations
- ☐ Extreme weakness
- ☐ Forgetfulness
- ☐ Memory loss
- ☐ Loss of normal logical thinking
- ☐ Insomnia or hypersomnia
- ☐ Loss of coordination
- ☐ Clouded thinking
- ☐ Exaggerated reaction to a stimulus (either too slow or too quick)
- ☐ Hallucinations (seeing, hearing, feeling, smelling, or tasting things that are not there)
- ☐ Tremors, spasms, or "the shakes" (mild to severe)
- ☐ Convulsions, seizures, or delirium tremens

Emotional Warning Signals

- ☐ Moodiness/mood swings
- ☐ Frequent crying
- ☐ Frequent guilt feelings
- ☐ Family problems
- ☐ Interpersonal problems
- ☐ Work-related problems
- ☐ Suicidal thoughts
- ☐ Homocidal thoughts
- ☐ Violent behavior

Medical Problems (Diagnosed)

Liver/Gall Bladder

- ☐ Hepatitis B (inflammation of the liver)
- ☐ Hepatitis C
- ☐ Cirrhosis (the second most common cause of cirrhosis, after alcoholism, is hepatitis C, which typically occurs among intravenous drug users)
- ☐ Cancer of the liver or gall bladder

Pancreas/Spleen

- ☐ Pancreatitis (inflammation of the pancreas)
- ☐ Cancer of the pancreas or spleen

Gastrointestinal

- ☐ Ulcers, recurring or nonhealing
- ☐ Esophagitis (inflammation of esophagus)
- ☐ Cancer of esophagus
- ☐ Gastritis (inflammation of the stomach)
- ☐ Inflammations of the intestines (colitis, Crohn's disease, and others)
- ☐ Cancer of the intestines, especially of the colon and rectum

Kidneys and Bladder

- ☐ Chronic bladder infections
- ☐ Cancer of the bladder
- ☐ Kidney failure

Nose and Throat

- ☐ Rhinitis (inflammation of the lining of the nose)
- ☐ Nasal mucous atrophy (thinning of the nasal lining)
- ☐ Sinusitis (inflammation of the sinuses)

Metabolism

- ☐ Hypoglycemia (low blood sugar)
- ☐ Diabetes (hyperglycemia: an excessive amount of sugar in the blood)

Lungs

- ☐ Bronchitis
- ☐ Pulmonary edema (excessive fluid in the lungs)
- ☐ Frequent pneumonia
- ☐ Lung abscesses
- ☐ Cancer of lungs

Cardiovascular

- ☐ Hypertension (high blood pressure)
- ☐ Thrombophlebitis (infection of the veins)
- ☐ Myocardiopathy (disease of the heart muscle)
- ☐ Endocarditis (infection of the heart valves)
- ☐ Congestive heart failure
- ☐ Stroke

Blood

- ☐ Anemia (deficiency of red blood cells that causes extreme weakness and sometimes fainting)

Joints, Muscles, and Bones

☐ Osteoporosis (loss of bone mass, causing bones to become brittle)

☐ Gout (inflammation of joints caused by imbalance in uric acid metabolism)

☐ Myopathies (various diseases of the muscle)

Eyes

☐ Various inflammations of the eye

☐ Lateral nystagmus (jerking movement of eyes with gaze to the left or right)

Sex Organs

☐ Male impotence

☐ Frequent urinary tract infections

☐ Various inflammations of uterus

☐ Amenorrhea (lack of menstrual period)

Skin

☐ Abscesses

☐ Cellulitis (infections under the skin)

Immune System

☐ Suppression of immune system functioning (caused by most drugs of abuse, including marijuana)

☐ Autoimmune deficiency syndrome (AIDS)

General

☐ Sepsis (spread of infection throughout the body)

Vitamin Deficiency Diseases

☐ Malnutrition

☐ Neuritis (inflammation of the nerves; most common: peripheral neuritis, which affects nerves in the limbs)

☐ Beriberi (nervous disorder due to lack of vitamin B1)

☐ Pellagra (disease caused by vitamin B3 deficiency that leads to skin eruptions, problems with digestion, nervous system disturbances, and eventual insanity)

☐ Scurvy (disease caused by vitamin C deficiency that leads to bleeding gums, serious internal bleeding, and extreme weakness)

Psychiatric and Nervous Disorders

☐ Neuropathies (any of various disorders or diseases of the nervous system)

☐ Panic disorders

☐ Convulsive disorders

☐ Degenerative nerve diseases

☐ Brain abscesses

☐ Organic brain syndrome (mental disorder involving disruption of thought processes; symptoms include impairment of judgment, memory loss, disorientation, agitation, and confusion)

☐ Major depression or depressive disorder

☐ Manic-depressive disorder

☐ Schizophrenia

You might have one or more of these problems. The more of these problems you have, the more you stand to gain by quitting drugs. When you quit the drugs, your body begins to heal itself. If these conditions haven't gotten too serious, you can improve them, if not heal them completely.

WILL YOU NEED INPATIENT CARE?

Withdrawal from some drugs is serious business. For example, the depressants cause dangerous side effects during withdrawal. In fact, withdrawing from a moderate to heavy habit of depressants can be life threatening. If you have this kind of habit, you almost certainly will need a medically supervised program when you withdraw. This usually requires a six- to-12-week period during which you methodically step down your daily dose.

Also, you might need to start your program with a short, three- to seven-day stay in an inpatient setting, or you might do better by spending two to four weeks at an inpatient treatment center. Many variations are possible.

Many people also go to inpatient treatment for withdrawal from heroin, and some go for cocaine or amphetamine withdrawal.

One of my clients, Jamal, had a 20-year heroin habit. He had tried to quit many times on his own but kept going back to the needle. Finally, in desperation, he went to the local hospital and told them that he was suicidal and that he needed to come down off heroin. They admitted him, helped him through detoxification, and then transferred him to a 28-day inpatient drug rehabilitation center. Jamal completed that program and, when he got out, began saying, "I feel too good. I don't want to go back to using." That was more than a year ago, and during this time he hasn't had one slip. Also, his relationship with his family has improved by leaps and bounds, and he was recently promoted to a manager's job where he works.

Jamal decided that he needed inpatient care to help him quit. What will you decide? You must determine ahead of time how severe your drug withdrawal will be and whether you'll need inpatient care when you quit. A doctor who is familiar with addictions can tell you whether you'll need inpatient care. Ask the doctor you have chosen to give you your checkup. However, if you don't go to a doctor, and *if you're in doubt,* the answer is *Yes, you will need inpatient care when you quit.*

You know your drug use better than anyone does. Do you begin to have serious physical and mental problems whenever you stop using for more than a day? If so, plan to use an inpatient center for detoxification.

Look around. Hundreds of centers are available. You can probably find four or five near you. Check each one, and ask questions about how they operate. Then pick the one that you feel is right for you.

When you go, plan to participate with the staff and other patients. You'll learn a lot by doing so. And when you go, take this book with you. That way you can continue to develop your own successful program for quitting. The remainder of this book contains hundreds of suggestions that will help you do this.

YOUR EVALUATION OF THE PROBLEMS

In the last chapter, you learned how you deny many of your problems related to drug use. So far in this chapter, you've searched inside yourself to identify some of these problems. You also had a thorough medical checkup.

Now it's time to use the information you've gained—and to make sure that you don't deny anything.

Worksheet #3

Problems You'd Like to Avoid

Instructions. Here you'll find a list of problems not mentioned in previous sections. Check any that bother you. At the end of the list, in the blank lines, write down any health problems you discovered from your medical checkup. Also, be sure to include anything that you learned from your own inner search.

I want to avoid:

- ☐ Losing self-control.
- ☐ Taking too many risks. I could seriously injure or even kill myself in an accident; or, I could seriously injure or kill someone else.
- ☐ Dying younger. (Moderate to heavy drug users die at significantly younger ages than nonusers.)
- ☐ Violence. Drugs make me violent. I could hurt someone I love; or, I could hurt someone I don't even know.
- ☐ Becoming the victim of violence.
- ☐ Letting a child (children) become the victim of violence.
- ☐ Becoming overweight. I eat too much when high; or, The drug I use slows the metabolism, causing me to gain weight.
- ☐ Becoming underweight or malnourished. Because of my drug use, I don't eat enough; or, The drug I use depletes my body of vital nutrients.
- ☐ Fetal abnormalities. (Even moderate drug use while pregnant is likely to cause serious disabilities in your developing child. In fact, every one of the psychoactive drugs is fat soluble enough to cross the placenta and get into the body and brain of your baby. The best way to look at it is this: If you want to use, don't have a baby; if you want to have a baby, don't use.)
- ☐ Looking older than I am. (Excessive drug use accelerates aging. The effects can be seen on the skin.)
- ☐ Problems with sex.
- ☐ Losing my sexiness. (In the male, many of the psychoactive drugs cause impotence, or the inability to get an erection; in the female, they cause orgasms to become weaker or to disappear.)
- ☐ Feeling like I'm a failure.
- ☐ Tension or anxiety.
- ☐ Mental confusion. I can't think clearly; or, I can't make up my mind about things.
- ☐ Feeling bad about myself.
- ☐ Feeling too dependent on a drug.

- ☐ Feeling too dependent on other people.
- ☐ Hurting my ability to love. (Drugs destroy loving relationships.)
- ☐ Feeling lost.
- ☐ Feeling lonely.
- ☐ Feeling that I don't have any sense of spiritual connection with the world.
- ☐ Losing good friends because of my drug use.
- ☐ Planning too much of my life around drugs.
- ☐ Feeling like I'm losing my mind.
- ☐ Losing memory. (Many of the psychoactive drugs cause neural damage, which leads to memory loss.)
- ☐ Feeling too much pain and physical discomfort.
- ☐ Fighting for control of my life.
- ☐ Dulling my sense of taste.
- ☐ Dulling my sense of smell.
- ☐ Depression.
- ☐ Nervousness.
- ☐ Paranoia.
- ☐ Feeling like I might commit suicide. (Drug users are five to 15 times more likely to commit suicide than nonusers.)
- ☐ Risking death by accidental overdose.
- ☐ Risking a serious reaction to an impure product. (Drugs made in clandestine labs often have impurities. Also, drugs are often cut with many, sometimes dangerous, products.)
- ☐ An irregular menstrual cycle.
- ☐ Infertility (women).
- ☐ A higher rate of miscarriage.
- ☐ Legal problems, or various drug-related arrests.
- ☐ Financial worries, caused by spending too much money spent on drugs and drug-related problems.
- ☐ Difficulty keeping a job.
- ☐ Losing self-esteem.
- ☐ Feeling like people don't care about me anymore.

- ☐ Feeling like everything is hopeless.
- ☐ Feeling irresponsible or immature.
- ☐ Feeling like I'm not taking care of myself.
- ☐ Getting angry too often.
- ☐ Feeling guilty or ashamed because of my drug use (or because of something I did after using too much).
- ☐ Feeling like the people I love are suffering because of my drug use.
- ☐ Lying about my drug use. I lie to others and even to myself.
- ☐ Denying that I have any problems from my drug use (even denying some of the problems in this worksheet).
- ☐ Feeling more stressed.
- ☐ Destroying my ability to work well.
- ☐ Being stuck in a struggle.
- ☐ Feeling exhausted or worn out.
- ☐ Messing up my sleep. (Many of the psychoactive drugs disturb sleep, especially REM, or dream, sleep.)
- ☐ Having the shakes in the morning.
- ☐ Having low energy or no energy.
- ☐ Staying addicted. The more I use, the more I want to use.
- ☐ Feeling as if I have no choice. Drugs take my freedom away.

Other drug-related problems I want to avoid:

- ☐ _____
- ☐ _____
- ☐ _____
- ☐ _____
- ☐ _____
- ☐ _____
- ☐ _____
- ☐ _____
- ☐ _____
- ☐ _____

Drugs cause these problems. However, drugs solve many of these problems as well, for example, tension, anxiety, depression, feeling stressed, feeling lost or lonely, and having no energy. How often do you use drugs to solve the very problems that drugs cause? Take another look at Worksheet #2: My Reasons for Using Drugs.

Drugs solve some problems, but they make the same problems get worse. This is called the "vicious cycle of addiction." From this point of view, using drugs seems like a tremendous waste of time. Why bother? All you gain is bad health and an early death. However, when you quit using, you break out of the vicious cycle, and, for the first time in years, you give yourself a chance to grow.

A new you, a solid you—a more interesting, nonaddicted you—begins to show itself. It gets stronger and stronger the longer you abstain from the drugs.

DO YOU WANT TO QUIT?

Now you can make a decision. It's a mighty task, weighing the benefits against the problems, but by this time, you have a good feel for it. What to do? Quit, or keep using? If you keep using, how long will you continue before you need to quit?

One thing for sure. If you keep using, you get fewer benefits and more problems. The life of a moderate to heavy user becomes nearly impossible. To get an idea of this, take a good look at some older users you know (or knew!) and imagine yourself in their place.

It's up to you. You might decide to quit using now, or you might decide to wait. Either way, Worksheet #4 will help. Your other work in this chapter has been leading to this one important list. When you quit using, you'll use this list over and over again.

Worksheet #4

Reasons for Quitting

Instructions. Any problems that drugs are causing become your best reasons for quitting. So, first, take another look at Worksheet #3.

On the following worksheet, instead of looking at the problems (the negatives), you'll see what you stand to gain (the positives). For example, instead of the problem "I'll die younger," here you'll note what happens when you quit using: "I'll live longer."

Here you'll see some good reasons for quitting. Check any reasons that you feel are important to you. Then, in the blank lines, write your own reasons for quitting. To do this, review the problems that you checked in Worksheet #3 and rewrite each problem to reflect a positive benefit you'll gain from quitting:

☐ I'll live longer.

☐ I'll get in control of my life.

☐ I'll be a more productive worker.

☐ I'll have more energy.

☐ I'll feel stronger at everything I do.

☐ I'll have better digestion.

☐ I'll greatly reduce my chances of getting hepatitis B, hepatitis C, or cirrhosis.

☐ My liver will begin to heal.

☐ It will help me cut down on tobacco.

☐ It will help me get things done more quickly.

☐ I'll feel more relaxed.

☐ I'll be able to think more clearly.

☐ I'll set a good example for my children.

☐ I'll have more time.

☐ I'll have more money.

☐ I'll feel happier.

☐ I'll feel liberated, free to do what I want.

- ☐ I'll gain self-confidence.
- ☐ I'll feel more mature.
- ☐ I'll feel like I've finally started making smart decisions.
- ☐ I'll regain my creativity.
- ☐ I'll become healthy. I won't feel as sick all the time.
- ☐ I'll have a better voice and a stronger, clearer throat.
- ☐ It will improve my nerves. I'll stop feeling nervous and tense.
- ☐ I'll be able to show my good qualities more often.
- ☐ I'll feel stronger emotionally.
- ☐ I can start healing. My body will repair most of the damage drugs have done.
- ☐ I can reduce my high blood pressure.
- ☐ I can avoid pancreatitis.
- ☐ I can avoid kidney damage.
- ☐ I can avoid _____(any other serious health problem that concerns you).

Continue your reasons for quitting by rewriting problems from Worksheet #3:

Now do one last thing. Rank your reasons for quitting in order of importance to you. Just put a "1" in front of the reason that's most important to you, a "2" in front of the next most important reason, and so on.

What are your seven most important reasons? Write them here:

1. _____
2. _____
3. _____
4. _____
5. _____
6. _____
7. _____

I suggest that you write these on a 3 x 5 file card and carry them with you everywhere. Review them whenever you feel the urge to use.

PART TWO

PLANNING YOUR OWN PERSONAL APPROACH TO QUITTING

CHAPTER 5

What About Narcotics Anonymous (NA)?

To be social is to be forgiving.
                    —*Robert Frost*

Have Friends. 'Tis a second existence.
                    —*Baltasar Gracian y*
                    Morales

Narcotics Anonymous (NA) was founded in 1953 by drug addicts who wanted to recover from addiction. They developed NA on the basis of the AA (Alcoholics Anonymous) model, which had already been tested with alcoholics. AA had been helping alcoholics quit drinking since 1935.

NA offers social support based on a model of religious fellowship. Members help one another stay clean and sober. At meetings, members talk about their problems and gain guidance from one another. Each member also works through the Twelve Steps, which give the recovering addict a set of goals (members call themselves "addicts"). Some of the steps offer moral and ethical corrections to help you turn your life around. Others help you find peace in God or gain strength through God "as you understand Him."

The Twelve Steps of NA are the same as those for AA, with only two minor changes: (1) AA's Step 1 reads, "We admitted we were powerless over alcohol. . . ;" NA's Step 1 reads, "We admitted that we were powerless over our addiction. . . ." (2) AA's Step 12 reads, ". . . we tried to carry this message to alcoholics. . . ;" NA's Step 12 reads, ". . . we tried to carry this message to addicts. . . ."

On the basis of a 1993 survey, the NA World Service Office estimates that there are 20,000 NA groups in the United States. If each NA group averaged 20 members, current membership would be about 400,000.

Today, NA is among the most recommended treatments for people who have problems with drugs. In fact, the Twelve Step format has become so popular that many look-alike programs have sprouted in the past 20 years. Aside from AA and NA, other programs, using the same group methods and similar 12 steps, include the following:

Overeaters Anonymous

Gamblers Anonymous

Alanon (for family members of alcoholics)

Alateen (for teenage family members of alcoholics)

ACOA (Adult Children of Alcoholics)

Sex Addicts Anonymous

Cocaine Addicts Anonymous

Indeed, NA can be a successful method for quitting drugs. Many have used it. However, if NA is as successful with addicts as AA is with alcoholics, its overall success will be limited. In the United States, about 5% of the recovering alcoholics use AA.

Of course, if NA is right for you, it can work wonders. In this chapter, you'll decide whether NA is for you. If it is, you can plan to use it as one of the methods in your approach to quitting.

On the other hand, if you happen to be among those who don't feel comfortable with NA or who don't like its methods, you needn't waste your time with it. In this book, you'll find many alternatives that will work for you.

HOW NA CAN HELP

NA can help you in many ways. In addition to those already mentioned, here are some others:

1. NA offers you total involvement in a community of nonusers. This makes it easier for you to break away from your total involvement with drugs. When you join NA, you join a ready-made social scene that can replace the drug scene.

2. As an NA member, you gain an important sense of belonging. When you belong to a valued organization, you feel more valued inside yourself.

3. Group members lend mutual support for not using drugs. This can be very helpful. As a popular song says, "We all need somebody to lean on."

4. It's easy to make new friends in NA. You'll have something in common with everyone you meet.

5. NA destigmatizes drug addiction. You're seen not as a "good-for-nothing dope fiend" but as someone with a disease. More important, it's not your fault.

6. NA helps you regain responsibility. You're not responsible for your disease, but you are responsible for maintaining your sobriety. It's up to you to stay away from drugs. You'll find that this new sense of responsibility will help you immensely.

7. In any treatment, you first need to accept your problem with drugs before you can begin to change. NA helps you accept your problem with drugs. The method works well for many people. You start by admitting your problem in front of the group: "Hello. My name is _____, and I'm an addict." Then, in Step 1, you admit your problem to yourself.

8. You can count on it. Meetings are held at many different times of day, seven days a week. Also, once you've started, you can find a sponsor. This is someone who's available for you 24 hours a day, seven days a week.

9. It's free, or it's available for a small donation at each meeting. This could be very important to you. Other treatments can cost thousands of dollars, and if you don't have health insurance, you might not be able to afford them.

Practice #2

Try a Few Meetings

Instructions. Try at least five NA meetings. First, get a schedule of different meetings in your area. You can have a schedule sent to you by calling your local phone number for NA. (If you can't find a local number for NA, call the national headquarters at 818-773-9999 to ask for a local listing.) Then select a few local meetings and begin going to them.

If you like the first group you go to, keep attending that one. If you don't like it, shop around. Each NA group has a personality all its own, and it might take a while to find one you like.

Make notes if you want. It helps many people to write about their experiences. You can write your ideas and your feelings about NA in your notebook.

Important rule: Don't go to the meetings while you're high on drugs. It's not fair to anyone, especially yourself. If you don't have a break in your drug use long enough to go to a meeting, wait until after you quit using, then do Practice #2.

DRAWBACKS TO NA

Many treatment professionals and many people who've tried NA have specific complaints about the organization's methods and beliefs. Here's a list of the most common criticisms:

1. NA neglects the physical. You get no medical advice and no information on healing. You get no encouragement to exercise, change your diet, use relaxation or stress-reduction techniques, or any helpful methods—other than NA. In fact, you might think that NA was encouraging *bad* health habits. At many meetings, sodas, cookies, cakes, or doughnuts are served, as are coffee and tea. Of course, both sugar and caffeine increase anxiety and nervous tension, especially in recovering drug users, who tend to have heightened reactions to these substances. (Note: In recent years, some meetings have changed.

Now you can find some meetings whose members are knowledgeable about health and that serve only healthy foods and beverages. You can also find a few meetings that are nonsmoking.) This is perhaps NA's biggest weakness. Even if you use NA, you'll do much better if you also use other techniques to help you heal the physical problems drugs have caused.

2. NA requires social involvement. You gain help by becoming part of a group. However, what if you're the type of person who gets nervous in groups? In that case, NA can feel like a major punishment. Many people use drugs to help themselves in social situations, to help them feel calm around others. Yet, NA forces you to be around others without the drugs. Facing this prospect, you might get terribly nervous.

Many people who try NA find that being in a group makes them want to get high—and that's what many of them do as soon as the meeting is over. If meetings cause this kind of anxiety in you, you might find it difficult to gain any help from NA.

(There's another related problem. A few of my clients have reported that pushers go to some of the meetings and try to sell drugs when the meeting is over.)

3. NA requires a specific religious belief. You must believe in God or some greater power. Otherwise, you'll be lost. Six of the 12 steps refer to God or a greater power. In these six steps, you must turn yourself over to God, admit things to God, ask God for help, and seek God through prayer or meditation.

NA allows some flexibility in beliefs. "God" can be "as you understand Him." Still, you might have difficulty with a certain defined concept of God. For example, you might not see God as a "Him."

Before quitting drugs, users often find that their strongest religious belief concerns "God, the Almighty

Drug." Many have given up their faith in "God, the Father" long ago. If, when you quit drugs, you can renew your belief in some kind of God, NA might be of help. However, if you don't fit NA's religious beliefs, don't worry. You can use any of the various spiritual or religious alternatives mentioned later in this book.

4. NA insists that you call yourself an addict. You might be a lot of interesting things, but at every meeting—if you speak—you must start by saying, "Hello. My name is _____, and I'm an addict." This reminds you, over and over, of a problem you have—not something good about you, but a problem. This negative reminder can help some people stay away from the problem (drugs), but it forces some to feel too guilty too often or to feel just plain stuck. At one meeting, you might like to hear everyone get up and say something positive, such as, "Hello. My name is _____, and I feel excited, happy, and refreshingly new today."

5. Many people have difficulty with the "public confessional" approach of NA. At meetings, members confess their problems with drugs. This might be helpful if it didn't take so much time every meeting. Stories about past problems have been called "war stories." You'll hear details such as, "The worst things I did while high on drugs . . ." or "How bad an addict I was. . . ." Too many of these stories make for a mighty dreary meeting.

In addition, you'll hear members complain about how difficult things are now that they're not using. You'll hear about "how much I wanted to use today when the boss yelled at me," "how terrible I have felt," "how I've had a tough time fighting the urge to use all day," and other complaints.

You might prefer more emphasis on the positive. Once again, if members dwelled more on the powerful, positive notes of their recovery, meetings could be much more uplifting.

6. NA fosters too much dependency among its members. It's like trading one addiction for another. You no longer depend on drugs but on NA. The new habit—going to meetings—beats the old habit in many ways, but some folks have difficulty giving so much of their lives to the group. After going to NA for a few months, one member said that she felt "completely controlled by the group," as if she were losing her identity. This problem with NA will be greatest among independent-minded persons.

7. For NA members, drugs remain the central focus in their lives. Before NA, members were preoccupied with using. In NA, they're preoccupied with not using. Now, instead of remembering the good old days, they remember how bad things were. Members recall problem after problem as they discuss the evils of drugs. This means that they cannot break their relationship with drugs. It's a love-hate relationship, but instead of leaving the relationship completely, they simply shift their involvement from love to hate.

8. NA members believe that you're powerless over your addiction. Is this true? It might be true before you were able to quit the drugs, but don't you show some power over addiction after you quit? Don't you show even greater and greater power over drugs the longer you stay away from them?

9. NA takes too much of its members' time. The hours you spend at NA every week you could be spending on some other positive or healthful activity.

IT'S YOUR CHOICE

You've gone to a few meetings. You know some of the good points about NA. You also know most of the reservations you have with NA. So now you can make a decision.

Worksheet #5

My Decision About NA

Instructions. On the left side of this worksheet, write what you like about NA. On the right side, write what you don't like. Write each statement in your own words.

What I like about NA   What I don't like about NA

_____   _____
_____   _____
_____   _____
_____   _____
_____   _____
_____   _____
_____   _____
_____   _____
_____   _____
_____   _____
_____   _____
_____   _____
_____   _____
_____   _____
_____   _____
_____   _____
_____   _____
_____   _____

Now evaluate your feelings and make a decision whether to join NA. If you're still not sure, try a few more meetings. Check one of the following four boxes:

☐   I like NA. I have no problems with it, and I will use NA when I quit.

☐   I like NA. The problems I have with it don't bother me that much, so I will use NA when I quit.

☐   I like some things about NA. But the problems I have with it bother me too much. I will not use NA when I quit.

☐   I don't like NA. I have too many problems with it. It will make things much harder for me, so I've decided not to use NA when I quit.

This is your decision. You can always change your mind later if you need to. No problem. But you've made up your mind for now. *So go with it.*

CHAPTER 6

How to Break a Habit

Habit, n. A shackle for the free.
          —*Ambrose Bierce*

Wise living consists perhaps less in acquiring good habits than in acquiring as few habits as possible.

          —*Eric Hoffer*

Everyone has habits—big habits, small habits. Some people have only a few habits. Some people have many.

In one sense, habits make life a little more convenient. Certain things seem easier. With just one way to do something, there's no need to think or to find a new way to do the same thing each time you approach it.

The problem is that you can get stuck in a rut. The more you do things by habit, the less adventure you have in your life and the less room for creativity. Too many habits or one very serious habit can chain you down. You can lose your sense of freedom. In fact, it can get to the point where you feel you're not doing anything new, just doing everything over and over by memory.

ALL ABOUT HABITS

What is a habit? A habit is a behavior that you repeat again and again. Once you learn a behavior that helps you in some way, you tend to repeat it. Soon it becomes a normal behavior for you. After a few repetitions, it becomes habit.

Here's how a habit begins:

1. You find a certain way to do something.

2. It works (it accomplishes your goal or solves some problem for you).

3. You stick to it (you repeat the behavior over and over).

4. You stop looking for other ways to do the same thing (there may be many other ways to accomplish the same goal, but why look for them now?).

Habits develop for good reasons, otherwise you wouldn't repeat the behavior. Even bad habits develop for good reasons. For example, in Chapter 4 (Worksheet #2), you looked at some of the good reasons you have for using drugs.

On the other hand, all habits cause some problems. Bad habits get worse, especially addictions. The longer you stay stuck in a bad habit, the more problems it causes. For example, in Chapter 4 (Worksheet #3) you determined what personal problems your drug habit causes. Even good habits cause problems. For example, you might develop the good habit of exercising. However, when you must do the same workout the same way each day or else feel miserable, you lose some freedom. In a sense, you relinquish some control over a part of your life.

Of course, the good you gain from the habit of exercising far outweighs the drawbacks. However, with a habit of using drugs, the good you gain dwindles, and the problems it causes begin to rule your entire life. Clearly, if you could simply exchange the habit of using drugs for the habit of exercise in your life, you would be doing yourself a magnificent favor.

Back to Basics

A habit is something you do in the *same way* each time you do it. The more you vary the way you do something, the less of a habit it is. Furthermore, a habit is usually the *only way* you use to accomplish a certain goal.

Habits can be *simple* or *complex*. Complex habits come in two kinds. The first combines many simple habits and can be called a *routine* or a *ritual*. The second kind of complex habit is based on a long-standing, deeply ingrained pattern of behavior. This kind of complex habit is the most difficult to break. Here are some examples of simple habits:

Putting on your clothes in the same order all the time

Combing your hair in same way all the time

Brushing your teeth

Taking a shower

Shaving

Putting on makeup

Doing the dishes, mowing the lawn, or doing some other household chore the same way every time

Sitting in the same chair for every meal or every time you watch television

An example of a complex habit that's a combination of simple habits is your morning ritual, or how you handle all the things you need to do each morning. For example, you might get up at the same time each workday, have coffee, take a shower, shave or fix your hair, get dressed, have breakfast, brush your teeth, and leave for work at about the same time. You perform each of these tasks in the same way, and in the same order, each day.

Examples of complex habits that are long-standing and deeply ingrained are the following:

Eating habits: These include not only the way in which you eat food (to see this, try eating with chopsticks or with your fork in your other hand) but also the foods you eat. Habits for certain foods run very deep, which is why most people have great difficulty changing their diets. Each of us tends to eat the exact same foods week after week. When we don't eat these foods, we tend to eat the same amounts of specific ingredients. This holds true for the amounts of salt, fat, protein, carbohydrates, and the total number of calories we consume. Each person has his or her own unique set of food addictions.

Personality: What we call personality is really an individual's *habitual* way of acting, a long-standing pattern of behavior.

Posture: This means holding your body in a certain way, carrying yourself in a certain way, usually favoring the same style over and over again.

Sexual behavior: Sexual compulsions and other unique sexual behavior appear to be deeply ingrained habits. Excessive or unusual sexual behaviors have been called "sexual addictions."

Emotional behavior: Each person has a deeply ingrained pattern for dealing with stress. Most of us tend to use the same reaction every time we have a problem—and to use this reaction instead of trying to solve each problem separately. A person's common reaction could be anger, violence, crying, whining, complaining, or becoming silent.

Addictions are the same as deeply ingrained, complex habits, but they take only a short time to develop. You can become addicted to most substances in less than a year. Some addictions take less than a couple of months to develop. All the drugs of abuse listed in Chapter 1 are examples of addictive substances. Others include sugar (sugar addiction might be considered a very powerful food addiction, but withdrawal from it looks more like drug withdrawal) and alcohol (actually two addictions rolled into one: sugar and a sedative drug).

Addictions change your biochemistry quickly and dramatically, which is why they become so powerful. All your cells, especially your nerve cells, crave the addictive substance. Without the substance, you start "climbing the walls." You might feel angry, nervous, depressed, sleepy, and even a little crazy when you try to withdraw from the addictive substance.

To one degree or another, all habits are difficult to quit. Even breaking a simple habit takes care and concentration.

BREAKING HABITS, MAKING CHANGES

Here are five steps to help you break a habit:

1. Know that you can change.
2. Unlearn learned behavior.

3. Make a decision to change.
4. Cope with cravings (or compulsions).
5. Find something to replace the habit.

If you follow these steps, you can break any habit. Now here's a detailed look at each step:

Step 1: Know That You Can Change

When you know that you can change, you can. Confidence is everything.

This seems like such a simple thing, but many people believe that they can't change. They have convinced themselves of this. They believe that the way they are is the only way they can be. So, right from the start, they're stuck.

This belief is just not true. Everyone can change. Anyone can change. You can, too. You can change any habit if you put your mind to it.

Millions of serious drug users have quit using. They found it hard, but they stayed with it and they were successful. You can be successful, too.

As you learn what to do, you'll become more and more confident. So show your confidence, and show your strength. You can make no greater demonstration of strength in the world than by quitting a serious addiction.

Step 2: Unlearn Learned Behavior

Habits are learned. You learn that certain behaviors help you in certain ways. The more you think a behavior helps you, the more you tend to repeat it.

For example, you might have a habit of crying (or complaining) because it helps you get your way. You might use drugs because it makes some of your problems seem easier to deal with. But remember: Any behavior that can be learned can be unlearned.

What does it mean to unlearn something? It means that you find another way to accomplish the same goal. You find another behavior (instead of crying or complaining) to help you get your way. You learn other ways to cope with life's problems (instead of using drugs).

Any habit can be changed. Some habits are easy to change, others are more difficult. In Practice #3, you'll break a few habits. When you do this, you'll see what it takes to unlearn a habit.

Meanwhile, if you haven't already quit using drugs, start considering how you'll break this habit. Whenever you use, remind yourself that you would rather not be stuck in an addiction for the rest of your life. Your drug habit doesn't fit in with your long-range plans. You're going to change. You're going to learn something new. You don't want to continue your excessive use of drugs. Soon you'll quit completely! Remind yourself that you would rather have better health, look better, feel better, live longer, think more clearly, deal with your problems more maturely, and finally feel liberated.

During the next few weeks, think of ways to deal with your problems *without using drugs,* and think of things that you could be doing instead of using. For example, what things would you like to do if your drug habit didn't take so much of your time? What things do you miss when you're messed up on drugs?

For the next few weeks—whenever you use— think of the things you miss. Later in this chapter, you can list them in Checklist #2.

Step 3: Make a Decision to Change

How do you make a decision to change? Keep three points in mind:

1. Want to change: This means that your heart is in it. The more you want to do something, the stronger your decision will be to do it.

2. Take responsibility for yourself: Take responsibility for any problems that you cause by your habit. When you take responsibility for what you do, you can break a habit. (Remember, too: Take responsibility for any new behavior that replaces your habit. It gives you a chance to feel proud.)

3. Have a clear goal or a clear set of goals: For example, when quitting their drug use, most people have two main goals: getting themselves free and regaining good health.

With these three points, you can turn your decision to quit using into an ongoing commitment and your new lifestyle into a welcomed joy.

Step 4: Cope with Cravings (or Compulsions)

A habit is something that you feel compelled to do. Even when you quit the habit, you still feel compelled to do it. If it's a habit related to food, drugs, or alcohol, you have cravings when you quit. If it's a habit related to a behavior, you have compulsions to repeat the behavior.

Addictions consist of cravings and compulsions. When you quit, you crave the addictive substance and feel compelled to use it again. For a while after you quit, your cravings and compulsions get stronger. Why? Your body wants to re-create the addiction-induced equilibrium. Over time, your cravings and compulsions diminish as your body adjusts to a new equilibrium.

To quit any addiction successfully, you need to cope with your cravings and compulsions. Probably the single best way to cope is simply to wait them out.

How do you do this? Each time you have a craving or compulsion, don't act on it—rather, simply be aware of it. Watch how it operates in your mind—and wait. While you watch and wait, your relaxed awareness will free you from the craving in a short amount of time.

What can you do during this period of time? Try continuing whatever activity you were involved in. Try deep breathing. Try exercise. Try any of the relaxation techniques in this book. Drink water, fruit juice, club soda, or herb tea. Eat a healthy snack such as carrot or celery sticks, popcorn, nuts, fruit, dried fruit (raisins or prunes), corn chips, or rice cakes. Try doing any of your alternatives to using drugs (see Checklist #2 in the next section).

When you first quit your drug use, your cravings are very strong. This means that you need to be just as strong to deal with them. But don't worry—you can do it. In this book, you'll learn many techniques that will work for you. Just be sure to use them.

And remember: The longer you stay away from the drugs, the easier it gets. Coping with your cravings does get easier. The main reason? You get stronger and stronger.

Step 5: Find Something to Replace the Habit

A habit helps you do a certain thing in a certain way. When you quit the habit, immediately you feel that something is missing. You find yourself with an empty space of time. You can fill this time in two ways:

1. You can find a new way to do the same thing.
2. You can do something completely different.

Let's look at these options:

1. Find a new way to do the same thing: For example, you might brush your teeth in a certain way every

time. When you break this habit, you can find a new way to clean your teeth. You can concentrate on a new method of brushing, change your pattern of brushing, or find some other way that doesn't include brushing, such as flossing with baking soda and rinsing with saltwater.

What about a drug habit? The drug helps you get high. When you quit it, you can find other drugs that will help you get high, but then you get addicted to these drugs. The solution? Find other (nondrug) ways to get high. Exercise works wonders. Relaxation techniques work, too. Even changing to a healthy diet helps you get high as you gradually regain the "glow" of good health.

There's another way to look at it. The drug habit helps you do many different things (see Worksheet #2). When you quit the habit, you can find new ways to do any of these important things. You can find new ways to calm down, new ways to socialize, new ways to have fun, and new ways to cope with certain problems.

2. Do something completely different: When you break a habit, you can use the time to do something else. If you choose this option, you abandon the habit as well as the goal of the habit.

When you quit using drugs, you give up the goal of the habit—getting high—and you gain hours and hours of extra time. In fact, you gain so much extra time that this can become a problem in itself. You might feel as if you have too much time on your hands.

So, when you quit using, you want to occupy yourself with other things you like to do. The more the better. Choose things that you now miss because of your using.

Maybe you would like fishing, building models, drawing, writing, doing anything artistic, redecorating your home, doing something enjoyable with your kids, or taking a class.

Soon after stopping the drug use, you'll find many new ways to enjoy yourself. But for now, practice breaking a few habits and see how you do.

Practice #3

Pick a Few Habits and Break Them

Instructions. Pick a few of your habits and break them. Use the list below to make your selections.

Here you'll learn to break habits and gain the confidence that you can change your life. For simple habits and routines, you'll learn to change the pattern of your behavior. For stronger habits and addictions, you'll eliminate the behavior completely.

When breaking a habit, pay close attention to what happens inside of you. Notice your consciousness. If you don't remain conscious of what you're doing, even for a brief moment, you tend to slip and fall back into the same pattern. So stay alert. Notice also what works for you when dealing with cravings and compulsions. Make notes. Make sure that you remember what techniques work best. You will use the same techniques to deal with cravings and compulsions when you quit the drugs.

For this practice, pick one habit from the first group, one from the second, and one or two from the third. Plan to break each habit for at least three weeks.

Simple Habits

Pick one of these habits and break it:

☐ Putting on shoes and socks: If you normally put on right sock, right shoe first, try putting on left sock, left shoe first.

☐ Taking a shower: If you normally wash your hair first and work your way down, try washing your feet first

---

and work your way up. If you normally take showers, start taking baths instead.

☐ Shaving: Use a pattern different from the one you normally use.

☐ Combing hair: Comb your hair in a different way or in a different style every day.

☐ Cosmetics: Put your eye makeup on in a different way.

☐ Cracks in the sidewalk: If you normally avoid cracks in the sidewalk, start stepping on them.

☐ (Your idea): _____

Routines

Pick one of these routines and break it:

☐ Morning ritual: Do everything in a different order. Remember, you'll probably have to get up earlier. Or just do something *completely* different. Idea: Get up, run around the house a dozen times, come in through an open window, kiss everyone in the house three times each, write a few lines of poetry, then leave for work (oops, are you still in your pajamas?).

☐ Work routine: As much as possible, change your usual pattern. Notice how your creativity at work begins to rise.

☐ Evening ritual: Again, change your entire routine as much as possible.

☐ Exercise routine. Try changing your routine. If you normally do sit-ups, push-ups, and jumping jacks, try going for a long walk instead. If you normally go jogging, try aerobic dancing.

☐ Watching television: This is a very strong habit; some call it an addiction. Try quitting completely. Do you feel freer? What can you do with all that free time?

☐ (Your idea): _____

Stronger Habits and Addictions

You'll find that these are much more difficult to break, so they give you better practice at quitting drugs. Pick one or two and break each for three weeks at a time (you can try recommended substitutes to help reduce cravings):

☐ Red meat, chicken, and eggs: Try substituting fish or bean dishes.

☐ Sugars: White sugar, brown sugar, molasses, honey, maple syrup, corn syrup, sucrose, glucose, dextrose, maltose, and fructose. These are very difficult to quit. Be aware of labels, as sugar is added to almost everything, even most brands of normal table salt. For craving, avoid chemical substitutes such as artificial sweeteners. Instead, try fresh or dried fruit.

☐ Dairy products: Milk, butter, cheese, and yogurt. When doing this, eat lots of dark-green vegetables, such as broccoli, kale, collards, and parsley. For cravings, try eating seeds and nuts, especially sesame seeds, sesame butter, peanut butter, and almond butter. The dark leafy greens are high in calcium, as are sesame seeds and nuts.

☐ White flour and white flour products: Substitute whole-grain flours, such as whole wheat or whole oat. Read labels, but be careful. If a label says "wheat flour," it's probably "white flour." It must say "100% whole-wheat flour" or "100% stone-ground whole wheat."

☐ Foods with chemical preservatives and artificial flavors: Another tough one. Read labels. Even when buying fresh fruits and vegetables, you're buying chemically sprayed or treated ones, unless the package says "organic" or "organically grown."

☐ Caffeine: This includes coffee, regular teas, cocoa, chocolate, cola (cola nut), some headache medicines, and many types of soda.

☐ Nicotine: This includes all tobacco products, a major addiction. If you can break your nicotine addiction, you can break any addiction.

☐ Alcohol: If you have a sizable habit, this will be difficult. If you are seriously addicted to alcohol, don't try quitting it casually. First get an assessment to see if you need inpatient care to help you with withdrawal.

☐ (Your idea): _____

WHAT ELSE CAN YOU DO?

Jump. Excite yourself. Ignite your mind with wonder, awe, and enchantment. Fill yourself to the brim with a lust for life. Utter unusual sounds. Envision waterfalls. Spin with vibrant, pulsing energy. Reel, rock, and roll.

Sit cross-legged on the table if you like. Do somersaults on the ground. Smile. Laugh out loud.

Do it all without drugs.

Some people ask, "When I quit using, what else can I do?" You can do a hundred different things. Two hundred different things. Anything you choose.

When you quit using, you open a whole new world. Instantly, you gain a great amount of time. At first you might be surprised at how much extra time you have.

Why does this happen? As a moderate to heavy user, you spend so much of your life preoccupied with drugs. When you make plans, you make sure to plan for the drugs as well. Sometimes you don't make any plans except for the drugs—you just know, whatever you do, you're going to be using. Sometimes when it's just you and the drug, you might feel that the drug is your only friend.

By quitting the drug use, you give yourself a great opportunity to do some different things—things you might miss doing now. With the extra time you gain, you can find many new and interesting ways to enjoy life, to overcome problems, and to realize goals. So, when you quit, it's important to make sure that you find some new things to do or new ways to enjoy the things you do already. The more alternatives you have to using drugs, the more exciting your life becomes.

In addition, your alternatives help you cope with cravings. They can help you cope with an immediate craving or help you when you're feeling tense. Some alternatives that take more time can seem like a total adventure away from drugs.

An alternative for you might be something as simple as doodling on a piece of paper for a few minutes or as complex as planning, and then taking, a special vacation. (By the way, when you quit the drug use, you'll be able to save enough money in one year to afford a really fine vacation.)

So just remember that whenever you feel a craving to use, do one of your favorite alternatives. Quickly, you'll forget about the craving.

What are your favorite alternatives to using drugs?

Checklist #2

Alternatives to Using Drugs

Instructions. Which alternatives would you enjoy doing? Look these over and put a check next to any one you would like to do. You can also write your own choices at the end of each category. (Remember too, that if you associate any of these with your drug use or, if it's something that you do while using, it might not be a good alternative for you when you quit.)

Now go back over the list and pick your favorites. Put a second check next to any alternative that you would *really* like to do.

When you quit the drug use, any one of your alternatives gives you a new way of enjoying life. But do your favorite ones first. It'll be more of a treat.

One other thing: Don't start doing any of these until after you quit the drugs. In that way, it will feel like a reward for quitting.

Creative Hobbies and Crafts

☐ Drawing
☐ Writing

- ☐ Sculpting
- ☐ Painting
- ☐ Music
- ☐ Photography
- ☐ Finger painting
- ☐ Doodling
- ☐ Collecting (anything from bottles to baseball cards, whatever suits your fancy)
- ☐ Building models
- ☐ Needlecraft/sewing
- ☐ Knitting/tatting/crochet
- ☐ Macramé/weaving
- ☐ Ceramics
- ☐ Model railroading
- ☐ Woodworking/cabinetmaking
- ☐ Tole painting/decoupage
- ☐ Tie-dyeing
- ☐ Metalwork/tinsmithing
- ☐ Leatherwork
- ☐ Making jewelry

Physical Activities: Exercise

- ☐ Walking/hiking
- ☐ Jogging/running
- ☐ Hatha yoga/stretching exercises
- ☐ Tai chi/karate
- ☐ Swimming
- ☐ Rowing/rowing machine
- ☐ Canoeing/kayaking
- ☐ Bicycling/bicycle machine
- ☐ Snow skiing/waterskiing/skiing machine
- ☐ Surfing/windsurfing
- ☐ Trampoline

- ☐ Dancing
- ☐ Aerobic exercise classes
- ☐ Roller skating
- ☐ Ice skating
- ☐ Weightlifting/Weightlifting and conditioning machines
- ☐ Jumping rope
- ☐ Any exercise routine or workout

Physical Activities: Sports

- ☐ Any of the above exercises or training activities, if done competitively. List here: _____
- ☐ Tennis/badminton
- ☐ Racquetball/handball/squash
- ☐ Baseball/softball
- ☐ Volleyball
- ☐ Basketball
- ☐ Soccer
- ☐ Field hockey/ice hockey
- ☐ Golf
- ☐ Bowling
- ☐ Boating/sailboating
- ☐ Fishing
- ☐ Croquet/bocci

Activities That Give an Adrenaline Rush

- ☐ Mountain climbing
- ☐ White-water rafting or canoeing
- ☐ Ropes course (offered at some addiction treatment centers)
- ☐ Hang gliding
- ☐ Bungee jumping
- ☐ Skydiving

Home and Garden

- ☐ Any home fix-it or repair job
- ☐ Auto repair work
- ☐ Mowing the lawn
- ☐ Installing a fence
- ☐ Cooking a new recipe
- ☐ Redoing a room
- ☐ Planting flower beds, trees, or shrubbery
- ☐ Installing a rock garden, sidewalk, or patio
- ☐ Any home improvement (painting, redecorating, re-modeling)
- ☐ Gardening (a lot of work with a clear benefit: raising good food for your table)
- ☐ Farming ("large-scale" gardening—might include raising animals)

Intellectual Pursuits

- ☐ Teaching yourself something new
- ☐ Taking classes
- ☐ Getting a degree
- ☐ Reading a book
- ☐ Going to a museum
- ☐ Making plans to do something special
- ☐ Working on your own personal life plans (this book gives you ideas for making new plans for a changing life)
- ☐ Studying something you would like to know more about. What interests you: _____
- ☐ Teaching someone something you've learned

Spiritual

- ☐ Religious activities (church, religious events)
- ☐ Studying spiritual teachings

- [ ] Practicing meditation or prayer
- [ ] Taking time for self-reflection
- [ ] Working with any spiritual techniques to gain personal inspiration and enlightenment
- [ ] Working NA's Twelve Steps (the spiritual and moral backbone of NA)
- [ ] Taking a spiritual self-help workshop
- [ ] Reviewing your morality—determining what's right and wrong for you—and following it

Social and Emotional: Helping Yourself

- [ ] Spending more time with friends
- [ ] Spending more time with loved ones
- [ ] Improving the quality of your friendships
- [ ] Improving your loving relationships:
  - [ ] Couples workshops
  - [ ] Marriage counseling
  - [ ] Family therapy
- [ ] Working on getting rid of emotional problems:
  - [ ] Self-study with books
  - [ ] Workshops
  - [ ] Counseling or individual therapy
  - [ ] Group Therapy
- [ ] Learning stress-reduction and relaxation techniques
- [ ] Learning assertiveness (how to stick up for yourself without being too aggressive)
- [ ] Finding one new friend who doesn't use drugs
- [ ] Developing a whole new set of friends

Social and Emotional: Helping Others

- [ ] Doing something special for someone else
- [ ] Getting yourself on a program to do one kind thing for someone every day

- ☐ Doing volunteer work at hospitals or for local service organizations
- ☐ Being a Scout leader
- ☐ Being more helpful to others at work
- ☐ Joining NA (helping others overcome their problems with drugs)
- ☐ Becoming a Big Brother or Big Sister
- ☐ Working for VISTA or the Peace Corps
- ☐ Visiting an elderly relative or friend
- ☐ Giving to a charity or joining a charity group

Vacations, Games, and Entertainment

- ☐ Getting away from it all: a vacation, special trip, family outing
- ☐ Visiting a recreation center
- ☐ Going to an amusement park
- ☐ Special events: concerts, sporting events
- ☐ Going out to dinner
- ☐ Going to a movie
- ☐ Playing a game with family or friends: card games, board games, any kind of game
- ☐ Playing solitaire (if you can make it a lively enough game!)
- ☐ Working a crossword puzzle or any kind of puzzle
- ☐ Listening to music
- ☐ Reading a book or magazine
- ☐ Pampering yourself:
    - ☐ A hot bath or a long shower
    - ☐ A visit to the beauty salon
    - ☐ A shave at the barbershop
    - ☐ Cooking a meal that you really like
    - ☐ Buying yourself a gift
    - ☐ _____
    - ☐ _____

☐ _____

☐ _____

Work

☐ Getting better at your work (This will come naturally; when you quit your drug use, you'll have more energy for your work.)

☐ Starting a new business (choose something you can do very well)

YES, YOU CAN CHANGE

If you want to change something about yourself, how do you do it? What's the best way?

First, you need to know what part of you that you want to change. You need to understand it completely. Then, when you understand it completely, you can drop it completely. You can let the whole thing go.

With drug use, you need to understand the whole picture. What makes you want to use? Why do you use too much? How does it affect you? You need to know the benefits you get from using as well as the problems it causes. Then, when you quit using, you can drop the whole behavior—the benefits and the problems. Soon you'll find new ways to get the same benefits, and, of course, you'll enjoy getting rid of the problems.

Here's another way to visualize a major change in your life, such as quitting drugs: View your "drug-using self" as a whole other self, a part of you that you no longer want. Then, when you're ready to change, kill the old self, the drug-using self. Now you can watch a new self emerge, a new, interesting, non-drug-using self. It's like being born anew.

Many people who have quit their drug use look back at the time they quit as a time of rebirth—a time of total transformation. The butterfly emerges from its chrysalis, never to be a caterpillar again.

It's Your Decision

Look in the mirror. Is that the same person you saw in the mirror yesterday? Is it the same person you saw there a year ago?

You continue to change whether you like it or not. Every day you keep changing. You are not the same you that you were yesterday. Some of the cells that were you yesterday are dead and gone. New cells have taken their place.

You're not even the same person you were five minutes ago. Things change. You're continually becoming someone new, someone different from who you were before.

How can it help you to know this?

It helps to free you. It helps you to realize that you're not stuck. And when you're not stuck, that means you're free to change.

You keep changing anyway. No matter what, you continue to change. You can change for the better, or you can change for the worse. It's up to you.

CHAPTER 7

Healing Through Diet

*One cannot think well, love well, sleep well if
one has not dined well.*
              —Virginia Woolf

*It's a very odd thing—
As odd as it can be—
That whatever Miss T eats
Turns into Miss T.*
              —Walter de la Mare

Without a doubt, diet is the single most important
component of good health. It's miraculous how
much healing takes place when you change from a
poor diet to a healthy one. Think about it. Whatever
you eat and drink becomes an intimate part of you.
You swallow your food, and immediately your body
begins to assimilate it. Through digestion, you become one with what you eat and drink. Through digestion, your body gains important nutrients.

The nutrients in food form the building blocks of
life itself. You gain strength from food. The strength
of every cell in your body depends on the quality of

163

the food you eat. How can you enjoy high-quality health? Eat high-quality foods.

Another benefit: Your mental and emotional health will improve. Through good nutrition, you can dramatically strengthen your brain's biochemical functioning. A balanced diet will make you feel balanced and energized. Such a diet enables you to think clearly, act calmly, and deal effectively with stress.

When you quit drugs, you can do yourself a big favor by changing your diet. With a good diet, you can improve your emotional outlook and heal most of the physical damage caused by moderate to excessive drug use.

The process is gradual but amazing. As you get healthier, you begin to feel younger. You have more zest. You even begin to look younger. This goes on for many years after you quit the drugs. It's as if you add lost years back onto your life.

What's more, the better your diet, the more effective the healing you'll experience. It might take you a while to learn how to follow a healthy diet, but the effort is definitely worth it.

THE IMPORTANCE OF DIET

Consider your diet. Are you getting the nutrients you need? If you use drugs excessively, the answer is no.

When you use a drug more than a few times a week, you begin to have problems. Why? Drugs reduce your body's ability to absorb nutrients. Too much of a single drug or too many drugs in your diet causes malnutrition.

Most drugs put severe stresses on the liver, pancreas, gastrointestinal system, brain, and nervous system. Other organs are affected adversely as well. Over time, organs and organ systems begin to break down.

Meanwhile, as the organs break down, your addiction gets worse.

However, when you quit using drugs, you can change your biochemistry through diet. With a healthy diet, you can improve your body's nutrition, strengthen your metabolism, curb your cravings for drugs, and become strong and healthy again.

A MATTER OF BALANCE

Your body seeks natural ways to balance itself. When out of balance, your body craves whatever it needs to regain balance. That's why you crave certain foods at certain times. This applies to drugs as well. Some of your craving for drugs is due to your body's need to achieve internal balance.

Your body balances your food intake on two scales: contractive/expansive and acid/alkaline. Too contracted, the body will crave expansive foods. For example, if you eat too many meats (extremely contractive), your body will crave sweets, alcohol, or drugs (extremely expansive). If you eat too many sweets, drink too much alcohol, or take a lot of drugs, your body will crave meats, eggs, or salty foods. Therefore, when you quit an extremely expansive substance, such as alcohol or drugs, you'll find it easier to quit some of the extremely contractive foods in your diet as well.

On the other scale, if you have an internal acid condition, you'll crave alkaline foods. For example, people tend to put a lot of salt (alkalizing) on meat or eggs (acid forming). People tend to like something sweet (acid forming) with coffee (alkalizing). Vegetables (alkaline) balance grains, beans, or meat (acid forming).

These "natural cravings" help you eat the right foods to keep you balanced—not necessarily healthy, but balanced. The body begins having problems when you eat too many extreme foods. Like a pendulum, you swing from one extreme to another, making it almost impossible to stay in balance. It's like trying to balance a seesaw by stacking heavy rocks on each end when, really, all you have to do is stand in the middle.

Contractive/Expansive

Foods can be contractive or expansive. Basically, expansive foods open you up, and contractive foods block you up. The body functions best in a mildly expanded state, slightly open. Thoughts come freely, blood flows freely, and the body eliminates waste easily.

When you eat too many contractive foods, you feel uptight, hardheaded, and possibly paranoid:

Extremely Contractive Foods
Salt
Red meat (beef, pork, lamb, veal)
Eggs

Moderately Contractive Foods
Chicken and other fowl
Hard cheeses

Mildly Contractive Foods
Fish
Sea vegetables (Irish moss, kelp, dulse, wakame, hiziki, nori, agar)

Other foods cause you to feel expansive. If you have too many of these foods, you get spaced out, confused, and possibly out of control:

Extremely Expansive Foods

    Drugs

    Alcohol

    Vinegar

    Sugar (all types, including honey and maple syrup)

Moderately Expansive Foods

    Fruit

    Dairy food (milk, soft cheeses, yogurt, butter)

    Nightshades (potatoes; tomatoes; eggplant; green, red, chili, sweet, paprika, cayenne peppers)

    Most herbs and spices

Mildly Expansive Foods

    Vegetables (most varieties except nightshades)

    Seeds and nuts

    Beans

Some foods are almost evenly balanced for expansive and contractive qualities. These are centered foods. They help you remain centered:

Whole wheat

Brown rice

Whole oats/oatmeal

Barley

Whole rye

Corn/cornmeal

Millet

Buckwheat

Acid/Alkaline

Strong blood is mildly alkaline. The alkaline blood is strong because viruses and other bacteria can't live in it.

Most people in the United States have acidic blood because of a diet high in acid-forming foods (mainly meats and sweets):

**Acid-Forming Foods,
from Most Contractive to Most Expansive**

>   Meat (all meats, including chicken and fish)
>   Eggs
>   Whole grains
>   Beans (dried, cooked)
>   Refined grains (white flour, white rice)
>   Seeds and nuts
>   Oil
>   Sugar (all types, including honey and maple syrup)

**Alkalizing Foods,
from Most Contractive to Most Expansive**

>   Salt
>   Fresh beans
>   Sea vegetables
>   Vegetables
>   Nightshades
>   Fruits
>   Fruit juice
>   Coffee

**Buffers (Partly Alkalizing, Partly Acid Forming),
from Most Contractive to Most Expansive**

Soy sauce and miso (fermented soybean products)

Tofu

Cheeses

Butter

Milk

Finding Balance

It's fairly easy to balance your diet on the acid/alka-
line and the expansive/contractive scales. Simply stop
eating too many extreme foods.

Cut out meats and sweets, and cut out alcohol and
drugs, including nicotine. Cut out or cut back on coffee. Cut back on salt. Cut back on oils. Cut out high-
cholesterol fats and oils. Cut out eggs. Cut out or cut
back on dairy foods. Cut out soft drinks. Cut out or
cut back any refined, processed, or partial foods, such
as white flour (breads, pastas, pastries, desserts), white
rice, lunch meats, and any products with sugars,
chemicals, or preservatives added.

Increase the amount of whole grains, beans, vegetables, fruits, fish, seeds, and nuts. Sound familiar? This
diet has been shown, in study after study, to be the
best for maintaining optimum health. This is the diet
recommended to avoid or decrease the risk of cancer.
It's the same diet recommended to reduce cholesterol
and the risk of heart disease. This diet will bring high
blood pressure into normal ranges. This diet heals
arthritis. This diet will control, and possibly cure, hypoglycemia. It will heal, and possibly cure, most of the
ailments caused by using drugs (see Checklist #1).

In short, the centered diet—as outlined on the next few pages—offers you the quickest, most complete way to heal yourself. Try it and see.

RECOMMENDED FOODS AND BEVERAGES

Whole Grains

Highly recommended. One of the most balanced foods you can eat. The body's natural digestion slowly breaks down the complex carbohydrates of whole grains into simple carbohydrates, or food for the cells. This slow process gives the body steady energy for a few hours.

Eat cooked whole grains as much as possible. Gram for gram, you'll gain the most energy from these. Otherwise, eat ground whole grains in bread, crackers, pancakes, and rolls—or even occasional desserts made with barley malt or rice syrup instead of sugar. You can also eat whole grains in the form of rice cakes, popcorn, and puffed wheat.

Whole grains should comprise 45% to 65% of your diet. Eat them as the main course for nearly every meal:

> Brown rice (short, medium, and long grain; basmati rice; sweet rice; other varieties; also prepared in rice cakes)
>
> Barley (pearl barley)
>
> Millet
>
> Whole oats (steel-cut oats, rolled oats, oatmeal; also roasted rolled oats in unsweetened or barley-malt-sweetened granolas)
>
> Whole wheat (cracked wheat, bulghur; also 100% whole-wheat bread, whole-wheat noodles and

pastas, puffed wheat, whole-wheat pastries and desserts)

Corn (corn grits, cornmeal, polenta; also cornbread, corn chips, tortillas, popcorn)

Rye (whole rye; also whole-grain rye breads, 100% rye crackers)

Buckwheat (buckwheat groats, kasha; also buckwheat noodles and buckwheat flour for pancakes)

Beans

Highly recommended. A fairly balanced food, slightly expansive, high in protein. Beans, when combined with whole grains, offer a complete source of balanced protein.

As you decrease the amount of meat in your diet, you need to increase the amount of beans. However, eat small portions compared to the whole grains in your meal.

Beans should form 5% to 20% of your diet. Eat small portions once or twice a day:

Chickpeas (garbanzos)

Lentils

Aduki

Black soybeans

Black turtle beans

Kidney beans

Pinto beans

Split peas (green or yellow)

Navy beans

Great northern beans

Lima beans (dried)

Red beans

Black-eyed peas

Bean products (tofu, tempeh, soy milk, soy condiments such as soy sauce and miso, various
"natural burger" mixes using ground whole
beans or peas)

Vegetables

Highly recommended. Fairly balanced, slightly expansive. Vegetables provide one of the best sources of vitamins and minerals to revitalize the body. What's
more, the vitamins and minerals in vegetables are
easy for the body to assimilate.

Vegetables should make up 20% to 30% of your
diet, four to five servings a day. Of your vegetable intake, about 50% should come from green leafy vegetables, about 25% from root vegetables, and about 25%
from squashes and other above-ground vegetables:

Dark-Green Leafy

Collard greens

Kale

Mustard greens

Broccoli

Parsley

Scallions

Watercress

Dandelion greens

Chicory

Leeks

Turnip greens

Carrot greens

Daikon and other radish greens
Chives

Roots

Carrots
Onions
Radishes
Turnips
Rutabagas
Burdock
Daikon radish
Lotus root
Parsnips

Above Ground

Squash (acorn, butternut, pumpkin, hubbard, Patty Pan, yellow/summer)
Cabbage
Brussels sprouts
Chinese cabbage
Bok choy
Cauliflower
Mushrooms
Shiitake mushrooms
Celery
Cucumbers
Green peas
String beans (green, yellow/wax, purple, others)
Escarole
Lettuce (head, Bibb, endive)

Sprouts (grain, bean, alfalfa)

Sweet potatoes/yams (seek locally grown varieties)

Sea Vegetables

Highly recommended. Well balanced, slightly contractive. High in minerals, sea vegetables help the body build strength and stamina. This is an important food to help you balance your diet when cutting back on meat. It should make up about 5% of your diet. Eat small portions, maybe four or five times per week:

Wakame (alaria)

Dulse

Irish moss

Hiziki

Arame

Kombu

Nori

Agar (kanten)

Seeds and Nuts

Recommended in small quantities. Fairly balanced, moderately expansive. Both seeds and nuts contain great amounts of protein and natural oils. Sesame seeds are extremely high in calcium. Almonds are a good source of calcium as well. Eat small portions. Very good roasted.

Seeds

Sesame

Pumpkin

Sunflower

Nuts
Almonds
Chestnuts
Walnuts
Peanuts
Pecans
Filberts
Brazil, hazel, cashew, pistachio (generally avoid
these unless you live in a tropical climate)

Seed and Nut Butters
Sesame butter or tahini
Almond butter
Peanut butter
Sunflower butter

Fish and Fowl

Recommended for occasional use. Fairly balanced,
slightly to moderately contractive. In small quantities, fish and fowl can be highly energizing. Both are
high in protein, yet lower in fat than red meats. They
should make up about 5% of your diet. Include in one
or two meals per week.

Fish and Seafood
Bass
Carp
Cod
Flounder
Haddock
Halibut

Perch

Salmon

Scrod

Sole

Trout

Turbot

Whitefish

Clams

Mussels

Oysters

Scallops

Tuna (somewhat unbalanced; use only a few times a year, if at all)

Fowl

Chicken

Cornish hens

Duck

Goose

Turkey

Fruits

Recommended. Fairly balanced in small amounts. From moderately expansive for northern-grown fruits to extremely expansive for tropical fruits. Fruit helps clear the mind and open the body. However, if you eat too much fruit, you can feel spaced out.

Fruit juice lacks the fiber of whole fruit and is recommended only in very small quantities (one or two ounces a day). Too much fruit juice can weaken the intestines.

The rule of thumb for fruit is to eat whatever grows locally (within 200 miles of you) and to eat only when it's fresh and in season. If you live in the North, don't eat tropical fruit. Also in the North, local fresh fruit is not available through the winter, except for apples. Dried fruits, such as raisins, store well and can be eaten anytime.

Northern Fruit (Temperate Zone)
Apples
Apricots
Blackberries
Blueberries
Boysenberries
Currants
Cantaloupe
Cherries
Grapes (raisins)
Honeydew melon
Nectarines
Peaches
Pears
Plums (prunes)
Raspberries
Strawberries
Watermelon

Tropical Fruit
Lemons
Persimmons
Tangerines

Avocados

Bananas

Coconuts

Dates

Figs

Grapefruit

Mangos

Oranges

Papayas

Pineapple

Pomegranate

Milk and Milk Products (Dairy Food)

Not recommended. Fairly unbalanced. Moderately contractive (hard, salty cheeses) or moderately expansive (soft cheeses, milk, butter, yogurt, cream).

These foods are high in calcium but also high in phosphorous, which blocks the body's ability to assimilate calcium. You'll gain much better calcium absorption from dark-green leafy vegetables. Dairy foods are high in protein but also high in cholesterol-type fats. Some dairy products have been mechanically processed to reduce the fat: skim milk, 1% and 2% milk, and low-fat cheeses. However, these refined dairy foods should generally be avoided. They have been manufactured by removing the butterfat from whole milk. Without the butterfat, the assimilation of calcium decreases. Further, without the protein-splitting enzymes in butterfat, digestion of so-called low-fat dairy foods becomes labored and incomplete. You'll experience better digestion and better calcium absorption with the whole-milk alternatives.

Of all the people in the world, about two-thirds are allergic to dairy food. You might want to get tested to see if you're one of them.

It's recommended to completely remove dairy foods from your diet or to cut back considerably. One method of cutting back is to quit all dairy foods for five or six days at a time, allowing yourself to have them only a day or two each week:

Milk

Butter

Cheese

Yogurt

Cream

Buttermilk

Sour cream

Ice cream (not recommended)

Goat's milk and goat's milk products

Sheep's milk and sheep's milk products

Nightshade Vegetables

Not recommended. Fairly unbalanced, moderately expansive. Nightshade vegetables upset the body's calcium metabolism by causing a biochemical reaction that removes calcium from the bones and redeposits it, by way of the bloodstream, throughout the body. This causes inappropriate calcification in the joints, kidneys, blood vessels, and soft tissue, including brain tissue. Indeed, some specialists recommend quitting the nightshades if you have any inappropriate calcification in the body, especially arthritis, osteoporosis, or other bone disease.

Interestingly, most diets high in nightshades will also be high in dairy foods. Most likely, the dairy foods offset at least some of the calcium loss from the nightshades.

For this reason, consider quitting dairy foods and nightshades together. Quitting only one at a time might cause calcium imbalances:

Tomatoes

Potatoes

Eggplant

Peppers (green, red, sweet, hot, bell, chili, paprika, cayenne)

Tobacco (smoked or chewed, it causes imbalances as well)

Eggs

Not recommended. Unbalanced, very contractive. High in protein but very high in fat, especially cholesterol. It's a powerful, highly concentrated food. Eat only one or two a month, or none at all.

Oils

Recommended in small quantities for cooking or salad dressings. Fairly unbalanced, expansive. Unprocessed, unsaturated vegetable or seed oils can complement various foods and help with digestion. The following are recommended:

Unrefined dark sesame oil

Extra virgin olive oil

Unrefined light sesame oil

Pure expeller pressed safflower oil

Unrefined canola oil (should not be used for cooking)

Pure expeller pressed flax seed oil (should not be used for cooking)

Natural Sweeteners

Recommended in small quantities if you crave sweets. Fairly unbalanced, expansive:

Barley malt

Rice syrup (yinnie syrup)

Juices (apple and other juices can be used as natural sweeteners in cooking)

Molasses

Maple syrup (in very small quantities)

Seasonings in Cooking

You can vary the taste of foods by using different seasonings. You can vary the texture, the saltiness, the sweet and the sour, or add variety with herbs and spices.

Thickeners

Kuzu

Arrowroot (powder or flour)

Agar (kanten)

For Salty Flavor

Sea salt

Miso (fermented soy paste: very good for making soups or sauces; many varieties, each with a slightly different flavor; highly recommended)

Soy sauce

Umeboshi (salt-pickled plum)

For Sweet Flavor See the section: "Natural Sweeteners"

For Sour Flavor

Brown rice vinegar

Other naturally fermented vinegars

Lemon

Herbs and Spices The milder the better. Fiery hot and other extreme spices can cause an unbalanced condition. Fresh is best, but naturally dried herbs and spices are okay, too. Use small amounts:

Basil

Ginger (very good, especially fresh)

Cinnamon

Dill

Garlic (if mild)

Oregano

Curry (if mild)

Marjoram

Thyme

Bay leaves

Tarragon

Poppy seed

Caraway seed

Coriander seed

Dry mustard

Carob (for occasional use only; can be used as a chocolate substitute)

Table Condiments

Choose your table condiments to add flavor to your food and to increase its nutritional value. If using a prepared condiment, such as pickles, mustard, or mayonnaise, make sure that it contains only the highest quality natural ingredients (natural sweeteners, whole grain vinegar, and pure vegetable oils):

Naturally fermented pickles and pickle relish

Natural mustard

Mayonnaise (eggless)

Natural salad dressings

Horseradish

Sea salt

Gomasio (roasted ground sesame seeds and sea salt: nutty flavor; very good on cooked whole grains)

Furikake (roasted nori flakes, sesame seeds, and miso)

Powdered dulse

Daikon pickles (daikon radish fermented in soy sauce)

Sauerkraut (salt-fermented cabbage)

Umeboshi plum and umeboshi plum paste (Japanese pickled plum; tastes good with some whole grains and vegetables; also acts as a blood purifier; a single teaspoon can quickly heal certain ailments, such as muscle cramps and upset stomach)

Shiso leaf (beefsteak leaves fermented with umeboshi)

Dried shiso leaf powder

Tamari soy sauce (very salty; use sparingly at the table)

Black pepper/white pepper (for occasional use; can be ground fresh at the table)

Beverages

It will help if you balance your intake of beverages the same way that you would balance your intake of foods. How? By avoiding extremes.

The single best beverage is *water*. However, make sure to drink only pure water from a well or spring or filtered from the tap. Here are some other suggestions:

Grain coffee

Chicory root coffee

Kukicha (roasted bancha twig tea)

Noncaffeinated teas (roasted barley tea, mu tea, roasted brown rice tea, dandelion tea; for occasional use: mint tea, chamomile tea, wild berry teas)

Club soda/seltzer water (chemical-free only)

Mineral water (sparkling or nonsparkling)

Homemade vegetable juices (occasionally)

Soy milk (occasionally)

Almond milk (occasionally)

Fruit juices from locally grown fruit (occasionally, in small quantities)

Foods to Avoid

You should avoid the following foods because they cause too extreme or too unbalanced a condition. Eat these foods only one or two times per year or not at all.

Animal Foods

    Red meat (beef, lamb, veal, pork)

    Certain seafoods (bluefish, crab, herring, lobster, sardines, swordfish, roe, red snapper, any smoked fish, caviar)

Vegetable Foods These are too high in acids or too expansive:

    Artichoke

    Asparagus

    Beets

    Chard

    Okra

    Rhubarb

    Spinach

    Zucchini

Spices

    Cayenne

    Saffron

    Nutmeg

    Cumin

    Cocoa (chocolate)

Fruits and Nuts Any that are not grown locally (see previous lists).

Oils and Fats

    Cottonseed oil

    Palm/palm kernel oil

    Coconut oil

Margarine

Any processed oil, including all hydrogenated oils

Animal shortenings (lard, bacon fat)

Condiments

Most commercial mayonnaise

Most commercial salad dressings

Refined salt

Commercial vinegars

Brewers yeast

Catsup

Sweets and Sugar Foods (read labels)

Jams and jellies

Doughnuts, cakes, pies, pastries

Chewing gum

Ice cream

Most breakfast cereals

Most processed food (in cans and jars)

Most commercially prepared dry foods ("instant" foods, mixes, other boxed foods)

Most breads

Many frozen foods

Sugar (names of sugars to avoid in any product: granulated white sugar, powdered white sugar, brown sugar, turbinado sugar, raw sugar, sucrose, dextrose, maltose, fructose, lactose, glucose, corn syrup, corn sweetener)

Honey (natural raw honey is a better choice than any of the refined sugars)

Beverages

Alcoholic beverages

Soft drinks and sodas

Coffee

Commercial teas

Caffeinated teas

Any extremely aromatic herbal teas

Refined and Partial Foods

Any white flour product (white bread, white flour/semolina noodles and pastas, white flour, pretzels and crackers, white flour pastries)

White rice

Sugar (see "Sweets and Sugar Foods")

Vitamin and mineral supplements (except for special short-term needs described later in this chapter)

Chemicalized Foods

Any chemical additive (read labels)

Dyed and colored foods (unfortunately, you won't find dyes listed on product labels, as it's not required by law)

Artificial sweeteners (any artificial sweetener: saccharine, sorbitol, Aspartame, Nutra-Sweet, and so on. These deceive the body. From a taste signal, the body prepares to deal with real sugar. Then, in the process of digestion, the body discovers that it's dealing with a different chemical. The liver and kidneys are hardest hit, as they work overtime detoxifying this chemical from the blood.)

Herbicides and pesticides (When buying fresh fruit and vegetables, buy "organic" and "organically grown" whenever possible. That way, you steer clear of fresh foods that have been chemically treated in the growing process. These chemicals get into and under the skin of fresh foods and can't be washed off completely. Also, when buying squash, cucumbers, rutabagas, and other root vegetables, avoid those that have been waxed. Finally, don't buy "fresh" fruits and vegetables that have been irradiated.)

Drugs and Medications

Any over-the-counter medication (Aspirin, cold and flu remedies, antacids, laxatives, and decongestants treat symptoms only, not causes. Food is the best medicine. If you want to treat the underlying causes of your symptoms, change your diet.)

Prescribed medications (These also treat only the symptoms, but much more serious symptoms. After quitting illicit drugs, you need to get off any prescribed medications that can be addictive and do this as soon as possible. But don't stop taking a prescribed medication without a doctor's order or without being under a specialist's care. To find other options, consult other specialists: physicians, dieticians, holistic healers, and so on. With a dietary plan such as the one in this book and a specialist who knows your situation, you should be able to make a smooth transition.)

Any illicit drugs (Any of the illicit drugs, including marijuana, creates too extreme a condition. They cause you to crave all kinds of extreme foods and become impossible to balance with a wholesome diet.)

HEALTHFUL WAYS OF COOKING AND EATING

How you eat is almost as important as what you eat. How you prepare your food and how you approach your food can make a world of difference. Here are some suggestions.

Use Various Methods of Preparation

You can gain additional variety in your meals and create different tastes for your foods by using various methods of preparation.

You can prepare a single food many different ways. For example, with rice you can pressure cook it or boil it, and you'll notice taste differences between the two. Once cooked, it can be added to soup, stew, or salad; to bread dough or muffins for baking; to pancake batter for panfrying; or you could make a stir fry with vegetables or simply reheat the rice by steaming.

Here's a list to give you some ideas:

Use Regularly

Pressure cooking (best with whole grains, some bean dishes)

Boiling (with the lid on for grains and beans, without the lid for vegetables)

Panfrying/Sautéing (with a small amount of oil but no water; good for fish, pancakes, and vegetables, especially onion or other root vegetables or summer squash)

Stir-frying (brown the ingredients, add a small amount of water, and then simmer covered for a few minutes; good for vegetables, fried grains, or grain with vegetable dishes)

Steaming (good for vegetables, especially dark-green leafy vegetables, winter squash, or bush or pole beans)

Baking (good for squash, fish, vegetable casseroles, chicken)

Stews (the works: vegetables, grains and beans, even whole-grain noodles, and thickened with kuzu or arrowroot)

Salads (combinations of raw and cooked)

Soups (made mainly with vegetables, often with the addition of whole grains or beans; best if flavored with miso or tamari soy sauce)

Use Only Occasionally

Broil (fish)

Deep-frying (chicken or tempura vegetables)

Use the Best Cookware

When you use top-quality cookware, your meals will taste better and be healthier for you, too. As soon as possible, throw away any poor-quality cookware and go buy whatever you need.

What's best? Stainless steel and cast-iron cookware. Also very good are enamel-coated cast iron, enamel-coated stainless steel, earthenware, and Pyrex.

Avoid aluminum, any nonstick cookware, and copper. Every time you cook with these implements, some molecules from them get into the food, making it taste slightly metallic or "tinny" and putting stress on your body. These substances can reach toxic levels quickly. In the case of aluminum, the body has trouble eliminating this metal. It builds in the tissue and can cause long-term problems. For example, aluminum has been linked to Alzheimer's disease. Research shows that the brain tissue of those who have died of Alzheimer's disease has, on the average, four times the amount of aluminum as a normal brain.

When using cast-iron cookware, some of the iron gets into your food also. Major difference: The iron is good for you.

For the same reasons, don't store food in metal or plastic containers. Metal and plastic compounds can leach into your foods. Tests show that the polyvinyl chlorides (PVCs) in plastics can be dangerous to your health. For storing food, use glass, wood, or nonleaded ceramic.

Chew Well

Many Americans not only eat fast food, they eat food fast. Often we gulp our meals, hardly even tasting the food.

Unfortunately, this taxes our systems, resulting in poor or incomplete digestion and malabsorption of nutrients. The reason? Digestion begins in the mouth. Saliva mixes with food to start the long process of digestion. It's the first key ingredient in the breakdown of food. In addition, the more we break down the food with our teeth, the more complete our total digestion will be. When we chew well, food remains in the mouth longer, and more saliva is produced. That means that the body can absorb and use more nutrients for each mouthful.

You can improve digestion 100% if you begin to chew your food well. Some authorities recommend you chew every mouthful 100 to 200 times. I recommend you start with 25 to 50.

Or try this: Chew as much as necessary to thoroughly pulverize your food. The more liquid your food is when you swallow it, the better.

Ghandi said, "You must chew your drinks and drink your foods." You'll find every meal more satisfying when you do.

Eat Only When Hungry

Some people feel a craving to eat all the time, especially after quitting an addiction to drugs, tobacco, or alcohol. When you use these substances addictively, your body gets adjusted to excesses. When you quit one of these substances, you tend to fill the gap with food.

How do you break the habit of overeating? The best way is by retraining your body. Listen to your inner needs, listen to your body's true signals for hunger, and learn to pay attention.

Sometimes it helps to wait five or six hours between meals or to fast for a whole day. This can help you focus attention on your inner sensations of hunger.

Don't eat just because "it's time to eat" but only when you're hungry. You'll soon learn to distinguish true hunger from "addictive hunger."

When You're Hungry, Eat

When you feel hungry, truly hungry, you should eat. And don't wait too long.

Why this rule? It's because you're likely to experience low blood sugar if you wait too long between meals. This will cause nervousness. You might get fidgety or even get the shakes. You might get angry with yourself and people around you. You can experience headache, tension, and most every hypoglycemic symptom.

If you feel hungry, eat. Sometimes a small, healthy snack will do. If you're really hungry, eat a regular meal.

To control hypoglycemia, many health practitioners recommend eating six meals a day. How? Just plan your day to include six small meals. In practice, you can plan for three regular meals, three healthy snacks, and no sugar foods. With a plan like this, your blood sugar will remain at a more constant level all day long. That means that your emotions will remain fairly steady as well.

The six-meal-a-day plan works very well. Especially when you first quit using drugs—while your body is adjusting to a new diet—plan to eat many small meals each day. It will help you over the hump and help you make your initial adjustment to a life without drugs.

Relax When You Eat

Sounds simple, right? It might not be. Many of us spent our first 15 to 20 years in families in which a great amount of tension surrounded every meal. Now, whenever we begin to eat, even when we're alone, we feel uptight.

If you relax when you eat, your digestion will be much more efficient. You'll tend not to eat too much, and you'll enjoy your food much more.

How can you learn this? First, simply be aware while you eat. Eat slowly. Allow yourself to enter a calm and peaceful state. Second, use some special techniques. Any of the relaxation techniques discussed in Chapter 8 can help immensely.

Don't Eat Two to Three Hours Before Bedtime

Here's a simple rule that can help you sleep better and help you feel better the next day: Don't eat before bedtime, and don't get up to eat in the middle of the night.

The reason? In sleep, your bodily functions slow down. You digest food more slowly. So, if you eat soon before sleep, the food remains undigested for a longer period of time. How does this affect you? Because digestion competes with sleep, your sleep becomes more restless. What's worse, you might still feel full in the morning and fatigued before the day begins.

When you first begin to change, you'll probably find it difficult to avoid food for two to three hours before bedtime, but stay with it. It's a habit that you can change, and a peaceful night's sleep can be well worth the effort.

When You Eat, Don't Overeat

Perhaps as important as what you eat is how much you eat. When you eat too much, you strain all the digestive organs, especially the liver.

When you overeat, you tend to feel sluggish, tired, or sleepy. You can also feel irritable or tend to anger quickly.

Nonetheless, overeating can be hard to cure. Why? When you quit using drugs, overeating comes naturally. You might start eating excess food at meals and excess food between meals. What to do? Here are two ideas that might help:

1. Take your time: At every meal or snack, take your time. Relax. Chew well. As you eat, listen to your body. Listen closely. Your body will signal when it's had enough.

2. Practice eating less: What happens if you don't hear the signal or if, when you hear the signal, you've already eaten too much? In this case, practice eating a certain amount, for example, a normal meal with small to average servings. When you've finished this, stop. Don't go for seconds. Get up from the table and begin doing something else. After a few minutes, you'll forget about eating. Now how do you feel? Lighter? More peaceful? Stronger?

How much should you eat at any meal? It's up to you. Take time to learn your body's inner needs and what's best for you. On this subject, here's an old proverb from the Talmud that might help: "In eating, a third of the stomach should be filled with food, a third with drink, and the rest left empty."

TO SUPPLEMENT OR NOT TO SUPPLEMENT?

For 50,000 years of human history, we have gotten our essential nutrients from the food we eat, but now we have another option. Essential nutrients are available in the form of supplements.

What are supplements? Supplements, in pills or powders, offer concentrated forms of vitamins, minerals, proteins (amino acids), and other essential body-builders. Where do supplements come from? Food. Like white sugar and white flour, supplements are highly refined food products. Manufacturers start with a whole food and chemically or mechanically remove everything except the desired product.

The best source of nutrients is food. When you eat whole (unrefined) foods, you get the important vitamins, minerals, and proteins plus the fiber, carbo-hydrates, essential oils, and all-important enzymes to help your body digest and absorb the nutrients.

However, what if your body has been abused by years and years of unbalanced diet, heavy use of drugs, and malabsorption of nutrients? Certainly you'll need some time to adapt to health. It might take a few weeks or a few months before your body can begin absorbing essential nutrients from the food you eat.

So, as soon as you quit using drugs, you might try certain supplements to restore your vitamin and mineral levels. Like jump-starting a car, it can give your body a quick boost and get you back on the right road.

Once you reestablish your ability to absorb nutrients, you should stop using supplements. This might take only a few weeks. Then your body can begin doing the work that it was designed to do: gaining its nutrients from food.

Guidelines for Supplements

Vitamin C Vitamin C helps to detoxify the liver. Some treatment specialists recommend 4,000–5,000 mg a day. However, too much can cause its own toxic reaction. I recommend 500 to 1,000 mg a day. The RDA (recommended daily allowance) for vitamin C is 60 mg. For comparison, one medium stalk of cooked broccoli has 160 mg of Vitamin C, one cup of cooked cauliflower flowerets has 69 mg, one cup of cooked kale, collards, or turnip greens has 100 mg, and one cup of chopped raw parsley has 100 mg.

Silamarin Silamarin also helps to detoxify the liver. This extract of milk thistle has been shown to improve the liver's efficiency. You might try it as a supplement before every meal for the first two weeks. Then stop taking it or reduce intake to one meal a day or one meal every other day.

Glutamine Recommended by many researchers, this amino acid can curb the craving for alcohol, drugs, and sugar. If you want to try it, take 500 mg two or three times a day between meals.

However, like vitamins and minerals, amino acids work together. By artificially raising one, others will be depleted. This means that, while taking glutamine, you might find yourself craving various protein foods that contain glutamine in relatively low proportions compared to other amino acids.

As an alternative to taking glutamine supplements, you could increase your intake of foods that are high in this amino acid. Natural sources include whole wheat, carrots, radishes, and cabbage.

Dosages Moderate to excessive use of drugs depletes our bodies of minerals and vitamins (especially B vitamins), yet supplementing these can be tricky. Why? First, you can overdose on supplements. Too much of certain supplements can cause a toxic reaction. For this reason, you need to take low doses (or no doses) of vitamins A, D, and E. Second, vitamins and minerals work together. Too much of one will deplete the body's supply of another.

Some manufacturers have balanced the vitamins and minerals in their supplements to match the proportions of vitamins and minerals found in the body. These supplements are the best. Buy them in health food stores, not grocery stores or pharmacies. The health food store product will come in a base free of sugar, salt, starch, artificial ingredients, and additives.

For comparison, here's a list of all the ingredients you want and the approximate amounts of each:

Vitamin A, 5,000 IU
Vitamin D, 100 IU
Vitamin E, 100 IU
Vitamin C, 500 mg
Vitamin B1, 50 mg
Vitamin B2, 50 mg
Vitamin B3, 100 mg
Vitamin B6, 50 mg
Vitamin B12, 50 mcg
Folic acid, 0.4 mg
Pantothenic acid (vitamin B5), 100 mg
Biotin, 100 mcg
Choline, 100 mg
Inositol, 100 mg
Vitamin K, 10 mcg
Bioflavonoids (rutin, hesperidin), 100 mcg
Calcium, 100 mg
Chromium, 50 mcg
Copper, 2 mg
Iodine, 150 mcg
Iron, 18 mg
Magnesium, 100 mg
Manganese, 5 mg
Potassium, 100 mg
Selenium, 50 mcg
Zinc, 20 mg

You might want to try a vitamin and mineral supplement that includes all these ingredients for a few weeks to a few months after you quit the drugs. This will replenish depleted supplies and help your body relearn how to absorb vitamins and minerals. Then you can stop taking it and get all your appropriate nutrients from good food.

So What's Your Answer?

To supplement or not to supplement? If you take my advice, you'll supplement for no more than a few months while in transition from drug use to a whole-foods diet. Two exceptions: First, if you can't make the change to a whole-foods diet (and especially if you eat a lot of junk food), I recommend that you keep taking supplements. Second, I recommend that you start taking supplements before you quit the drug use and continue taking them until you make the change to a whole-foods diet. The diet of moderate to heavy drug users is about the worst there is and needs as much help as it can get.

If you don't like my advice, you can choose any of the following options.

Long-Term Supplementation. Some researchers and treatment specialists recommend the long-term use of supplements. For two approaches to this method, see the following:

> *The Hidden Addiction: And How to Get Free*, by Janice Phelps, M.D., and Alan Nourse, M.D. Boston: Little, Brown, 1986.

> *Eating Right to Live Sober*, by Katherine Ketcham and L. Ann Mueller, M.D. New York: New American Library, 1983.

Optional Short-Term Supplementation. Some authorities recommend this approach, which is similar to mine. See either of the following:

Food for Recovery: The Complete Nutritional Companion for Recovering from Alcoholism, Drug Addiction, and Eating Disorders, by Joseph Beasley, M.D., and Susan Knightly. New York: Crown Publishing, 1994.

Good Food for a Sober Life, by Jack Mumey and Ann Hatcher, Ed.D., R.D. Chicago: Contemporary Books, 1987.

No Supplements. Other specialists recommend no supplements whatsoever. See the following:

Food and Healing, by Annemarie Colbin. New York: Ballantine Books, 1986.

Healing Ourselves, by Naboru Muramoto with Michel Abehsera. New York: Avon Books, 1973.

HOW TO MAKE THE CHANGE

Get Into Cooking

You'll need to take some extra time with cooking. This might be a burden at first. However, with a little patience and perhaps a slightly different perspective, you can learn to enjoy it.

Remember to plan ahead. A bean dish from scratch (starting with dried beans) takes about two hours to cook. Whole grains usually take an hour. But here's the good news: You don't have to watch these dishes cook. Just check on them every half-hour or so. Also, if you make a big potful, it saves time. The next few days, you can reheat leftovers in minutes for many different dishes.

When you plan ahead, everything seems to take less time. At least you know what to expect and can accept it.

Overall, you'll probably spend more time preparing meals. You might even resent having to spend the extra time (I know I did), but here's a thought that helped me: For every hour I spent preparing healthy meals, I kept telling myself that I would gain an extra three hours on the total length of my life and that my life would be a healthier life as well.

Try Various Recipes

Starting a new diet can be viewed as a great adventure. So many new foods! So many new ways to prepare them! It's your opportunity to try as many new recipes as you can. For the first few months, try five to 10 new recipes or cooking styles each week. You'll enjoy the variety and become quickly proficient in the new diet.

Here are some recommended cookbooks with recipes for using whole foods and natural, healthy ingredients:

The Self-Healing Cookbook, by Kristina Turner. Vashon Island, WA: Earthtones Press, 1989 (good starter book).

Macrobiotic Cooking for Everyone, by Edward and Wendy Esko. Tokyo: Japan Publications, 1980 (good starter book).

Introducing Macrobiotic Cooking, by Wendy Esko. Tokyo: Japan Publications, 1983 (good starter book).

The Book of Whole Meals, by Annemarie Colbin. New York: Ballantine Books, 1983.

Deliciously Simple, by Harriet Roth (former director of the Pritikin Longevity Center). New York: New American Library, 1986.

The Vegetarian Epicure (two volumes), by Anna Thomas. New York: Alfred A. Knopf, 1978.

Still Life with Menu, by Mollie Katzen. Berkeley, CA: Ten Speed Press, 1988 (or try *The Enchanted Broccoli Forest* or *The Moosewood Cookbook*, also by Mollie Katzen).

The Ancient Cookfire, by Carrie L'Esperance. Santa Fe, NM: Bear & Company, 1998.

The Gradual Vegetarian, by Lisa Tracy. New York: Dell Publishing, 1985 (gives a great three-step method for making a gradual change from a meat-based diet).

Get Acquainted with New Foods

How do you get acquainted with new foods? Learn where to shop and what to look for.

Where to Shop Some supermarkets now carry whole grains, dried beans, organically grown produce, and other "health food" selections. Look for these sections in your supermarket.

Also, in most areas you can find health food stores and natural food cooperatives. Check them out. Many great selections are available at these stores, plus the workers there can be very helpful. Begin shopping at these alternative food stores for a good portion of your supplies.

Of course, if you live near any organic farmers, you might want to buy some of the foods that they grow and sell at roadside stands. Or grow your own. If you start your own garden, you can enjoy high-quality foods and get some exercise, too. A great combination!

What to Look For When you shop, read labels. Look for the very best ingredients: no chemical additives, no preservatives, no refined foods (such as sugar and white flour), and no artificial ingredients. Pay top dollar to get the best quality. Don't skimp on the food you eat. After all, the food you select will enrich your very life.

What If You Don't Like the New Foods?

At first, you might not like many of the new foods. That's natural. Whenever people make a major dietary change, they have the same problem. But after a while, you'll adjust to the new tastes and respond to new feelings aroused by foods.

With the new diet, keep reminding yourself that these foods will help you look younger, regain your health, and feel better. These reminders, in turn, will spark your desire to stay with the new foods.

Moreover, it doesn't take too long before you begin to taste the wholesome goodness of these foods. Give your taste buds a little time to adjust. Soon you'll find many favorite foods on the new menu—foods that you'll like as much, if not more, than your current favorite foods.

However, you might absolutely dislike certain aspects of this diet. If so, don't worry. You can choose another special diet.

With one caution: Choose a diet for health. Don't choose a diet for weight reduction. Why? Weight-loss diets tend to be extremely unbalanced in one way or another. In the long run, these diets can cause serious problems. Anyway, on a healthy diet, your body finds its own best weight, whatever is fit and trim for you.

Here are some healthy diet alternatives:

The Pritikin Diet: See *The Pritikin Program for Diet and Exercise,* by Nathan Pritikin with Patrick McGrady, Jr. New York: Grosset & Dunlap, 1973.

Raw foods diet to cure hypoglycemia: See *Hypoglycemia: A Better Approach,* by Dr. Paavo Airola. Phoenix, AZ: Health Plus Publishers, 1977.

Vegetarian: See *Transition to Vegetarianism,* by Rudolph Ballentine, M.D. Honesdale, PA: The Himalayan International Institute.

Or you can try one of these books on dietary cures for addictions:

The Hidden Addiction and How to Get Free, by Janice Phelps, M.D., and Alan Nourse, M.D. Boston: Little, Brown, 1986.

Good Food for a Sober Life, by Jack Mumey and Anne Hatcher, Ed.D., R.D. Chicago: Contemporary Books, 1987.

Eating Right to Live Sober, by Katherine Ketcham & L. Ann Mueller, M.D. New York: New American Library, 1983.

Need More Support?

Changing your diet takes a great deal of inner strength. Some people go it alone without any problem, whereas others do better with outside support.

If you need support, here are four places to look:

1. Start at home: Get your spouse, your family, or your roommates on your side. Explain that you're going to start eating healthy foods. Invite them to do the same. Tell them that they

too can gain greater strength, have more energy, and live longer, healthier lives if they'll join you.

Even then, you might not get too many takers. Just like you, they've become addicted to the foods they eat, and most people don't want to give up those foods, no matter how much you try to convince them of the damage they cause.

So be prepared. You might have to go it alone at home. Plan to make separate meals from your spouse, family, or roommates if they don't want to participate—but then watch how they continue to be curious about what you eat, and watch how you gradually win them over in the long run.

2. Try a support group: In most areas, you'll find various "natural foods" groups, such as Pritikin groups, vegetarian groups, and macrobiotic groups. These groups meet regularly, usually to share a meal and exchange good thoughts.

3. Try cooking classes: These are similar to support groups, except you'll meet in a kitchen. Here you can gain helpful hints on cooking and learn to make many interesting recipes.

4. Go to a dietary counselor: A dietary counselor will give you individual attention and a personalized diet to meet your specific needs. When you go, be sure to provide accurate information, for example, how long you've been using drugs, what kind of health ailments you have, and what kind of foods you eat.

When selecting a nutritionist, make sure that he or she steers away from any refined or processed foods. Also, make sure that this nutritionist doesn't advocate the "four food groups" classification system. Too many inconsistencies arise from this system. Of course, this system has now been officially replaced by the "food pyramid," which is a better system. It can bring you better health but, overall, only slightly better than the four food groups. The reason? The pyramid offers better guidelines for selecting foods, but it doesn't go far enough in eliminating poor-quality foods. You can gain better health from other types of diet.

Here are some suggested types of dietary counselors:

Holistic health practitioners
Macrobiotic dietary counselors (at East-West Centers across the nation)
"Whole foods" nutritionists
Pritikin health counselors

What About Dining Out?

When on a health-food diet in a junk-food world, dining out can be a nightmare.

The good news: You can now find more vegetarian and natural foods restaurants. Go to these as much as possible. Take a little extra time out of your schedule if necessary.

The bad news: It's not always possible to get to a good restaurant.

Solution: Get a salad. Even fast-food restaurants offer salads. Other possibilities are side dishes of vegetables (any cooked vegetables or coleslaw but not french fries), fish, chicken salad, or chicken (not deep-fat fried).

How to Begin a New Diet

Change Gradually, or All at Once? Which kind of person are you? Some people like to ease into things. Others prefer to make sweeping changes without looking back. For example, when quitting coffee, some people gradually decrease their consumption little by little over a period of months. Others simply can't decrease their consumption slowly. It's all-or-nothing for them. Even if they drink five to 10 cups a day, they need to quit it all at once—cold turkey.

What will be easiest for you?

Make a decision now concerning how to start your new diet. Gradually, or all at once?

When to Make the Change You can change some parts of your diet before you quit using drugs and change other parts later. If you want to make some changes before you quit using, here are the easiest things to do first:

Stop eating white-flour products and white rice; start eating whole-wheat products and whole rice.

Stop eating chemicalized foods: artificial flavors, artificial sugars, chemical additives, and preservatives.

Stop eating sweets and sugar foods. (To do this, you'll need to quit alcohol as well because alcohol converts to sugar in the body.)

Cut out nicotine.

Cut out caffeine. (Don't substitute decaffeinated coffees or teas. These products still contain some caffeine. What's worse, they're loaded with chemicals from the manufacturing process, with one exception: organically grown coffee, decaffeinated with the patented "Swiss water process.")

Add as many vegetables to your menu as you can, especially dark-green leafy vegetables.

(Note: You won't be able to change all of your diet *before* you quit using drugs. The reason? Drugs keep your diet too unbalanced. Drugs are so extremely expansive that you'll need strong contractive foods (meats, eggs, or salty foods) to balance them.

However, by changing some things before you quit using, you can get a head start on the new diet. This will help, especially if you are someone who likes to change gradually. Even if you prefer to change things all at once, you can view each category separately. For example, you can change from white-flour products to no white-flour products, you can quit coffee or cigarettes completely, or you can quit chemicals all at once.

Nevertheless, if you prefer to wait until you quit using the drugs and do *everything* at once, do that. This might be just the right approach for you.

HOW TO HANDLE CRAVINGS

What are cravings? What can you do about them? Can you ever cheat by having some of the food (or drug) you're craving?

What Are Cravings?

Cravings stir you. They nag you and try to cloud your mind. Cravings fight with you, attempting to control your behavior.

When you quit the drugs, you'll get cravings for them. When you quit sweets, you'll crave sweets.

Quit meats, and you'll crave them. When you quit anything that your body has adjusted to, you'll get cravings for it.

In the body, cravings are biochemical expectations. Each of us craves different things because each body has a biochemistry that is different from everyone else's. In part, you create your own internal biochemistry because it depends on the kinds of foods you eat and the kinds of drugs you take. Yet all human bodies are the same in some ways. For example, our bodies expect to get a certain set of biochemical nutrients from our diets. Take something away, and the body will notice immediately. It will "think" that it's missing something. This feeling inside, of something missing, is what we call craving.

Cravings can be of two kinds. You can crave things that your body needs (vitamins, minerals, proteins, oils, and carbohydrates from various sources), or you can crave things that you don't need (alcohol, drugs, and sweets and sugar foods).

Both kinds of cravings depend on the body's biochemical expectations. For example, alcohol and drugs raise dopamine, serotonin, or endorphin levels in the brain, biochemically causing calmness, pleasure, or euphoria. The body craves the alcohol or the drug on the expectation that pleasurable sensations will follow each time. Now let's take a look at the other kind of craving. Let's say that you drink orange juice frequently and that orange juice in your diet has become a primary source of vitamin C. This means that whenever your body needs vitamin C, you'll begin craving orange juice. If your body had been accustomed to getting vitamin C from broccoli and dark-green leafy vegetables, whenever your body got low on vitamin C, you would begin craving these particular vegetables.

Now imagine what it would take for you to change. Could you teach your body not to crave the orange juice when needing vitamin C and to crave the broccoli and dark-green leaves instead? Try it. You'll notice that it takes a long time for the body to learn this replacement.

That's why staying on a new diet can be so difficult. The body keeps craving foods from the old diet. This craving will persist until your body adjusts to gaining its essential nutrients from the new foods.

A suggestion: When you quit the drugs, change to your new diet the same day. That way your cravings for food and for drugs get mixed. What's so good about this? Because food cravings tend to overcome drug cravings, you won't notice your drug cravings as much, and this makes quitting so much easier.

What to Do About Cravings?

For food cravings, stay with the new diet and wait them out. Give yourself some time. Often the body makes an adjustment on its own. While waiting, try this: When experiencing a food craving, consider what your body is telling you. Feel it. What does the body want? What food in the new diet might satisfy the craving? When you do this, you'll discover more about the inner workings of your body, and you'll learn what kind of foods are good for you.

For drug cravings, use any way you can to reduce your cravings for drugs. Use the dietary techniques you learned in this chapter and the exercise and relaxation techniques you'll learn in the next chapter.

Meanwhile, beware of other excesses. When you quit your drug of choice, you'll tend to fill in the gap with alcohol or other drugs, or you might start overeating. You'll tend to eat more sweets, smoke more cigarettes, drink more coffee, or take more over-the-counter medications such as aspirin. Avoid this tendency as much as possible. It will just keep you craving your drug of choice for a longer period of time after you quit using it.

Finally, the most important dietary changes to help reduce your cravings for drugs are to reduce your intake of animal protein (the less meat and eggs you eat, the less you will crave drugs) and to increase your intake of whole grains, fruits, and vegetables.

In general, simply stay with the new diet as strictly as you can. Gradually, your body will adjust to the new foods, and your cravings for various foods and drugs will diminish. Immediately, you'll benefit from greater nutrition. As this happens, you'll gain more strength, stamina, and willpower.

When to Cheat?

Can you ever give in to your cravings without compromising your health? Yes and no.

Yes, you can give in to food cravings under certain circumstances. No, you can't give in to alcohol or drug cravings.

Here are some guidelines: If cravings persist, wait at least a full two days for food cravings and a full four days for sweets cravings. Then, if you're still craving, allow yourself to have some, and enjoy it, like giving yourself a treat. But study it, too. Whether it's a steak or ice cream, you might notice, over time, that you begin liking these treats less and less.

Here's a special stopgap measure you can take when you crave drugs: Don't give in to a drug craving. Wait, do exercises, put it off another day, do more exercises, and wait some more. However, if you're having an outrageous craving for drugs, to the point where you can't control it, have a caffeinated beverage or something sweet.

The only problem is that in a couple of hours you'll probably get the cravings again. So don't use this method too often, or you reduce its effectiveness. Remember, caffeine and sweets are addictive, too. You need to quit these in order to improve your health and strengthen your nervous system. So, cheat with caffeine or sweets only under dire circumstances. If it's a matter of using a drug or having a half-gallon of ice cream, have the ice cream.

Practice #4

Start Your New Diet

Instructions. If you've already quit using drugs, start your new diet now. Get into it as quickly as you can but as gradually as you need to.

   If you haven't quit the drugs, you can start making some of the recommended dietary changes. Even if you don't make the changes immediately, take time to get the cookbooks and get acquainted with new foods and food stores—and begin planning. Plan to stop using drugs soon and to start eating for health at the same time.

CHAPTER 8

Building Inner Strength

Consciousness of our powers increases them.
—Vauvenargues

What's the single most important thing you can do after you quit using drugs? Return to health as quickly as possible. Why? Health means strength. By returning to health, you gain both physical and mental strength, and both kinds of strength will help you abstain from drugs.

As you become stronger, you become more aware, more sensitive. You gain the power to make more decisions. You actually gain consciousness. It's like a new awakening, a new dawn. Building your inner strength helps you build a powerful awareness of your true inner self.

How do you build your strength? The same way you build your health: through diet and exercise. With proper diet and sufficient exercise, you become strong and healthy.

However, anyone who has been a moderate to heavy drug user has much to overcome. Why? Because drugs take something from you. Instead of building inner strength, they tear your insides apart and deaden your consciousness. You might feel powerful when you're high, but it's a false power. When you come down, you feel nervous, depressed, and lost.

For those addicted to drugs, poor health is like a cloud surrounding you—a cloud that gets darker and darker. When you quit your addiction, the cloud slowly clears. As you regain health, you begin to see again. Everything appears fresh and new. There is probably no better feeling in the world than the feeling of regaining your health.

To be sure, good health acts as its own reward. Health brings happiness. The healthier you become, the happier you'll feel—and the less you'll want to fall into the pattern of using drugs.

So energize yourself. Renew yourself. Regain your health as soon as possible.

We've looked at dietary ways to improve your health. Now let's look at exercise. You can work with two kinds of exercise: physical and mental. Physical exercise strengthens your heart, improves your circulation, and gives you more energy. Mental exercise—changing your way of thinking—helps you manage stress, feel relaxed, and become more self-confident.

In this chapter, you'll discover how to do the following:

1. Energize yourself with exercise

2. Calm yourself with relaxation techniques

3. Improve your self-image with assertiveness skills

4. Reduce inner tension with stress management and coping techniques

5. Renew human caring through friendship

EXERCISE

Action is the proper fruit of knowledge.
                    —Thomas Fuller, M.D.

Physical exercise builds physical strength. With exercise, your muscles improve, your body tone improves, and your internal organs get stronger.

However, here's something you might not know: Physical exercise builds mental strength as well. It's true. Scientists have pinpointed a biochemical reason for this. Vigorous physical activity causes the body to produce endorphins, the body's natural tranquilizers, which act on brain cells and nerve cells. They calm you in the same way as morphine, a related chemical.

So, to find peace and calm when you quit the drugs, get into exercise. It has a naturally tranquilizing effect. Without physical exercise, you can become nervous and depressed, or your life can seem dreary and dull. Endorphins, however, create a natural high. These powerful biochemicals can help you beat depression and stave off anxiety.

Tennyson once said, "I myself must mix with action, lest I wither by despair." This holds true for everyone. So when you quit the drugs, begin using the time you gain to become as active as possible.

How do you get active? Plan your own exercise program, one that will work for you. Then begin doing it.

Worksheet #6

Plan Your Own Exercise Program

Physical exercise not only helps build health and inner strength, but it is one of the most powerful tools to help beat depression. On this worksheet, you'll plan for two kinds of physical exercise: aerobic exercise and casual exercise. Make sure to add both to your personal program for quitting drugs.

AEROBIC EXERCISE

Aerobic exercise is highly active. It's a fast, physical workout that lasts 20 to 30 minutes without interruption. This kind of exercise strengthens your heart and circulation and leaves you feeling relaxed for 12 to 24 hours.

Aerobic exercise gives you the greatest production of endorphins, the body's natural tranquilizers. Perhaps you've heard of "runner's high." This describes the point in your workout when you begin to feel euphoric, usually after 20 to 30 minutes of vigorous activity.

You'll gain the greatest benefits by planning three or four aerobic workouts per week. Scientific studies show that the heart begins to lose the benefits of conditioning when more than two days go by without exercise. So, if you exercise on Monday, you'll need to exercise again by Wednesday and no later than Thursday to stay in shape and keep your heart fit.

When selecting exercises, be sure to choose those that match your way of life, those that are fun for you and easy to do. Also, keep in mind that you don't have to do the same thing all the time. You have many options. For example, let's say that you already play soccer on Saturdays. You could then plan a brisk walk for Mondays, go jogging on Tuesdays, and work out on the rowing machine in your basement on Thursdays.

By the way, it's a good idea to plan for four aerobic workouts each week. That way, if you miss one, you still achieve the minimum of three workouts. From the previous example, suppose that it was raining cats and dogs on Monday and you missed your walk. You still have your run planned for the next day, so you meet the minimum requirements. If it was pouring the next day, too, you can't let this day go by, so you can start jogging in place or go down to the basement and work out on the rowing machine.

Use the following checklist to choose your aerobic exercises. Then use the weekly schedule to plan a typical week. To qualify, all of the following must be done briskly for a minimum of 20 minutes without interruption:

Exercises

- ☐ Jogging/running
- ☐ Running in place
- ☐ Walking/hiking
- ☐ Swimming
- ☐ Rowing/rowing machine
- ☐ Canoeing/kayaking
- ☐ Bicycling/bicycle machine
- ☐ Cross-country skiing/skiing machine
- ☐ Trampoline
- ☐ Dancing (vigorous)
- ☐ Aerobic exercise classes
- ☐ Roller skating
- ☐ Ice skating
- ☐ Indoor workout and conditioning machines
- ☐ Jumping rope
- ☐ Any vigorous exercise routine or workout

Sports

- ☐ Ice Hockey
- ☐ Basketball (if you play a nonstop full-court game)
- ☐ Soccer
- ☐ Tennis (singles)
- ☐ Handball/racquetball
- ☐ Downhill skiing

Other Possibilities

- ☐ Mowing lawn (riding mowers don't count)
- ☐ Gardening (active phases such as hand-hoeing a row for planting, shoveling mulch)
- ☐ Splitting wood
- ☐ Shoveling snow
- ☐ Painting a room

☐   Trimming a hedge

☐   Your choice: _____

_____

Remember the main test for aerobic exercise: You must stay continuously active in the exercise for at least 20 minutes.

Develop a Weekly Schedule

Select four days of the week when you can schedule 30 minutes for an aerobic workout. Then select what time you'll do the workout. It can be a different time each day. Just make sure that you choose times when you are free. Write the times exactly. For example, on Monday you might want to work out in the morning, from 7:00 to 7:30, and on Wednesday you might choose the late afternoon, from 5:00 to 5:30. Now write in the exercise you'll do at these times. The first exercise you write will be your preferred exercise for that time. Then write in a backup exercise. This will be the exercise you'll do in case you cannot do your preferred exercise.

	Time of Day	Exercise	Backup Exercise
Mon	_____	_____	_____
Tue	_____	_____	_____
Wed	_____	_____	_____
Thu	_____	_____	_____
Fri	_____	_____	_____
Sat	_____	_____	_____
Sun	_____	_____	_____

One precaution about a 20- to 30-minute nonstop workout: You'll probably need to work your way up to such a long, vigorous workout. Start slowly and build your way up. If you have any soreness or any pains, especially chest pains, stop! Remember that it takes time to get in shape. Find your own pace and don't push yourself.

If you have any serious physical problems, you might need specific guidelines for exercise. Consult with your doctor. If you are 35 years old or older, make sure to have a medical check-up before you begin.

Give Yourself Time to Gain the Benefits

Although exercise brings about a natural high, it takes a while before you can feel this benefit clearly. You need to recondition your body to get it accustomed to training. You'll notice that the effects of exercise are cumulative. They get stronger the longer you've been at it.

It takes a while to break old patterns. The drugs you've been using create an instant high. If your body has become adjusted to drugs, all your cells have become lazy. Your cells get high without having to perform any activity. However, in the long run, this lethargy at the cellular level causes disease.

Activity brings health, so give yourself time. The benefits—euphoria and relaxation—come gradually but are well worth it.

Also, keep in mind that the high you get from exercise might not feel as high as the high you get from drugs, but the exercise high is solid. You don't feel spaced out or out of control. Plus the exercise high stays with you.

A Myth About Exercise

Many people feel that physical exercise wears you out. This is a myth that needs to be dispelled. Physical exercise actually gives you more energy throughout the day. The more you do, the more you can do.

By the same token, the less you do, the less you can do. If you lounge around, that's all your body will want to do. You'll feel more tired all the time. You'll actually need more sleep. You'll feel sick more often, and you'll get sick more often. Also, you'll feel depressed, often seriously depressed, most of the time.

If you want to put it to a test, try this: Work out for three days and see how you feel. Then lie around for the same amount of time and compare your feelings.

You'll notice that physical exercise doesn't wear you out. Rather, it improves your health, vitality, and energy.

Gaining Momentum

It might take you a while to build momentum, to get yourself to the point where exercise feels natural. But rest assured that it will happen. You might have to force yourself at first, but after a while you'll find yourself actually wanting to exercise.

Remember, the more you do, the more you can do. Your body adjusts. After a while your body gets into a rhythm and doesn't want to miss any of your workouts.

That's when you have momentum on your side. Once you get your exercise going on a fairly steady, regular basis, you tend to keep it going. So stay with your program long enough to get the momentum working for you. Then everything gets easier.

CASUAL EXERCISE

Any physical activity not vigorous enough or not long enough to be considered aerobic can be called a casual exercise. Our lives are filled with casual exercise. Just walking from room to room is a casual exercise.

The worst thing you can do is lie around. Why? You'll get depressed—and stay that way. It's a vicious cycle: Lying around makes you depressed, and what's the only thing you want to do when you get depressed? Lie around.

So don't get caught in this trap. Plan to be as active as you can. Instead of using your car, walk or ride your bike. Instead of using escalators or elevators, take the stairs. As much as possible, use your own human power instead of machines. Use hand saws instead of power saws, use push mowers instead of riding mowers, and wash the dishes by hand instead of using a dishwasher.

Also, plan to do stretching exercises, especially yoga. Yoga is just about the best all-around exercise you can do (for more details on yoga, see next section, "Relaxation Techniques").

Use the following checklist to choose your casual exercises:

☐   Stretching exercises

☐   Yoga

☐   Walking (short distances: two miles or less)

☐   Bicycling (less than 20 minutes)

☐   Any other aerobic exercise for less than 20 minutes

List:

☐ _____

☐ _____

☐ _____

☐ Nonaerobic sports

    ☐ Baseball

    ☐ Bowling

    ☐ Football

    ☐ Golf

    ☐ Volleyball

☐ Crafts

☐ Carpentry

☐ Gardening (all aspects)

☐ Work around the house (including normal housework: mowing lawn, raking leaves, vacuuming, cleaning, doing dishes)

☐ Repair projects (car and home)

☐ Weightlifting

☐ Gymnastics

Practice #5

Begin Doing It

Start your exercise program.

First, increase your casual exercise as much as you can and begin your weekly schedule for aerobics. Give yourself two months to adjust to the new schedule. After two months, plan to be following your weekly schedule exactly.

Your long-range goal? To make exercise an integral part of your life and to reap the rewards of increased health, peace, and happiness.

RELAXATION TECHNIQUES

The posture of the body is the posture of the mind made visible.

—Amrit Desai

What do you think of when you think of relaxation? Most people think of putting their feet up, lying back, and not doing a thing. But this is not relaxation. Why? When you remain inactive, nervous energy builds. This nervous energy needs to be released through activity before you can truly relax.

What kind of activity? Physical exercise works well (see the preceding section). It discharges tension and leaves you feeling relaxed. Some mental exercises also work well. In the next two sections, you'll learn certain mental practices that will help you reduce tension and manage stress.

In this section, you'll look at physical activities that reduce tension and relax you at the same time—during the activity. These specific techniques not only bring immediate relaxation but also leave you feeling relaxed for a long time afterward.

Here are the five most powerful relaxation techniques:

Yoga

Yoga is probably the most powerful relaxation technique. It serves as a complete physical exercise system.

It consists of many different stretching exercises, or poses, that you do in rhythm with your breathing. By breathing as deeply as you can, using your entire lung capacity, and moving as slowly as you breathe, your mind naturally focuses on the harmonious movement of body and breath. During this process, your blood is oxygenated and your heart rate becomes slow and steady. With each pose, you stretch your body to its muscular limit but never exceed this limit. Then, as you hold the pose and breathe as deeply as you can, the muscles you're stretching begin to relax. As they do, you release a tremendous amount of tension from your body.

You'll also notice how different poses massage and tone your internal organs. This helps to heal you. Moreover, the continued practice of yoga makes you feel integrated and at peace with the world.

To learn yoga, take a class with a local certified instructor or try any of these books to learn it on your own:

Integral Yoga Hatha, by Swami Satchidananda. New York: Henry Holt & Co., 1970.

Yoga for Your Life: A Practice Manual of Breath and Movement for Every Body, by Margaret D. Pierce and Martin G. Pierce. Portland, OR: Rudra Press, 1996.

Hatha Yoga: The Hidden Language, by Swami Sivananda Radha. Palo Alto, CA: Timeless Books, 1989. A workbook by the same author and publisher is available: *The Hatha Yoga Workbook.*

Lilias, Yoga and You, by Lilias M. Folan. New York: Bantam Books, 1972.

Light on Yoga (revised edition), by B.K.S. Iyengar. New York: Schocken Books, 1977 (highly advanced but perhaps the most definitive book on hatha yoga).

Also, try any one of these videos:

Let's Do Yoga, with Mimmie Louis. Redondo Beach, CA: Double Star Productions.

Health, Yoga and Anatomy, with Amrita Sandra McLanahan, M.D. Buckingham, VA: Integral Yoga Distribution (Satchidananda Ashram).

Lilias/Alive with Yoga (Volume 1 for Beginners), with Lilias M. Folan. Portland, OR: Rudra Press.

Deep Rhythmic Breathing

Deep rhythmic breathing relaxes your nervous system and energizes your body. Moreover, once you learn it, you can do it almost anywhere. Here's the basic method:

Lie on your back on the floor. Keep your legs straight or, if it feels more comfortable, pull your feet up until your lower back and the bottoms of your feet rest flat on the floor. Then place your hands on your abdomen, below your rib cage, so that you can feel the movement of your diaphragm.

Breathe in slowly, filling the bottom of your lungs (the area under your hands). Doing this, you should feel your abdomen rising and expanding. Then fill the midlungs (lower chest) and feel your rib cage expanding. Complete the inhalation by filling the upper part of your lungs as you feel your chest opening and rising slightly. Although these three phases seem separate, they occur in one uninterrupted movement, like a wave rising from your abdomen through your chest.

Now, breathe out slowly and evenly. Empty the bottom of your lungs first, feeling your abdomen flattening. Then empty your midlungs and then your upper lungs.

When deep breathing, begin each inhalation and exhalation at the abdomen. With each breath, feel the movement rising up through your chest from the abdomen as you fill or empty your lungs.

Practice breathing through your nose. Breathe directly into the back of your throat, partially closing your epiglottis, as if snoring faintly. When you breathe into the back of your throat like this, you open the passageways to your lungs. This produces a deep, resonant sound by which you can gauge the smoothness and evenness of your breath.

Think of the sound of each breath as a musical note that you're holding as long as possible (without running out of breath). This visualization will help you to breathe deeply and rhythmically. The deeper and more rhythmic your breath becomes, the more you'll relax.

Try taking 20 to 30 breaths each time you practice deep breathing.

You can also learn deep rhythmic breathing by taking a yoga class because yoga depends on coordinating bodily movement with the movement of your breath.

After you learn deep rhythmic breathing, you can do it almost anywhere. Even in social situations, you can take a few deep breaths and relax without being conspicuous.

Progressive Relaxation

Progressive relaxation is a way of controlling tension by first creating it and then releasing it. You can do this with your muscles. First you tense a group of muscles and then relax them. By systematically working your way through all the muscle groups in the body, you can relax your entire body.

Here's how:

Lie on your back with your arms and legs free. Start with your feet. Tense all the muscles in your feet, then relax them. Repeat two or three times. Now continue the same procedure with each muscle group, in this order: calves, thighs, buttocks, abdomen, chest, back, hands, arms, shoulders, neck, and face.

Next, tense all the muscles in your body at once, then relax. This will help you let go completely. Repeat this process a few times until your body feels loose and totally relaxed. Progressive relaxation is a quick way to get rid of anxiety and nervous tension. Try it and see.

Stretching/Warm-Up Exercises

Traditional American stretching exercises also relax you. Usually done as a warm-up and sometimes as a cool-down to a vigorous workout, these stretching exercises release tension from the muscles. For a good how-to book, try the following:

> *Stretching*, by Robert A. Anderson. Bolinas, CA: Shelter Publications, 1980.

Sex

Ever think of sex as relaxing? Well, it is, but not just any kind of sex.

Relaxation can be achieved after the long, gradual, lovemaking kind of sex. Experts estimate that it takes 30 minutes in the sexual embrace before we experience an actual chemical change inside our bodies. This chemical change has been linked to such positive benefits as the healing of internal organs and the reduction of tension. Complete relaxation washes over lovers after a long embrace.

(Important note: If you've been a moderate to heavy drug user, you might have health problems pertaining to sex. Also, you might need to reestablish a positive emotional relationship with your partner. So give your body and your emotions time to heal before trying this technique.)

For information on sexual techniques, see the following:

Sexual Secrets, by Nik Douglas and Penny Slinger. New York: Destiny Books, 1979.

The Tao of Love and Sex, by Jolan Chang. London: Wildwood House, 1977.

The Art of Sexual Ecstasy, by Margo Annand. Los Angeles: Jeremy P. Tarcher, 1989.

The Joy of Sex, by Alex Comfort. New York: Simon & Schuster, 1972.

ESO: Extended Sexual Orgasm, by Alan and Donna Bauer. New York: Warner Books, 1983.

Checklist #3

Relaxers: What Works Best for You?

Instructions. Try all the relaxation techniques just described. Then select two or three that work best for you. Check them on the list below and begin using them regularly.

☐ Yoga

☐ Deep rhythmic breathing

☐ Progressive relaxation

☐ Stretching/warm-up exercises

☐ Sex

ASSERTIVENESS TRAINING

When dealing with other people, do you remain on an even keel? Most people don't. We tend to overreact or underreact, at least some of the time. What happens when we behave this way? Our stress level increases.

At one extreme, you might blow up too often. You might yell or scream or get hostile with others.

On the other extreme, you might let other people run over you too often. You might become silent or overly agreeable or simply let other people get their way too often.

When you act too much on either extreme, tension builds and your relationships will seem distorted or incomplete. In one case, you force too much of yourself on others. In the other case, you give too much of yourself up.

However, there is a middle ground. Your behavior in your relationships can be both socially appropriate and emotionally fulfilling. This middle ground is like Baby Bear's porridge in the story of the three bears: It's not too hot, not too cold, but just right.

This middle ground is called assertive behavior; the extreme stances just described are called, respectively, aggressive and passive behavior. The more you act from the middle ground in your relationships, the better you'll feel. Assertive behavior means sticking up for your rights and protecting your needs—without overdoing it. It means that you don't let others push you around, nor do you push others around to get your own way. Let's look at an example:

Situation: You're waiting in a long line at the grocery store or the movies. Someone butts in line ahead of you.

Aggressive response: You get mad, raise your voice, and start yelling, "Hey you—get out of here! Get back to the end of the line where you belong!" After an incident like this, your anger and tension stay high for a long time.

Passive response: You don't say a thing. You get mad, but you keep it inside. Soon you get mad at yourself for being such a pushover, for letting people get away with such things. Your tension and internal stress remain high for quite a long time after the incident.

Assertive response: You go up to the person and say, in a normal tone, "I know you must be in a hurry, but we've all been waiting for a long time before you got here. Please go to the end of the line and wait your turn like everyone else." With this response, you do something to solve a problem. Even if the person wants to argue, if you remain levelheaded, that person will look like a fool.

You'll confront numerous situations every day that call for assertive behavior. A cashier might short-change you, a waiter might bring you the wrong order, or someone might jump in the door of the taxi you just hailed. These situations happen among strangers, but most problems with behavior transpire among friends, especially intimate friends. Among close friends, one person might yell to get her way, and another person might passively give in all the time. This is common. However, relationships like these remain immature. They do not grow, as they lack fairness. Partners in these relationships bully the other or allow themselves to be bullied. In either case, the relationship feels incomplete.

Which kind of person are you? Are you aggressive or passive? How can you become assertive? Here are some books that will help:

When I Say No I Feel Guilty, by Manuel J. Smith, Ph.D. New York: Bantam Press, 1975.

Your Perfect Right: A Guide to Assertive Living, by Robert Alberti, Ph.D., and Michael L. Emmons, Ph.D. San Luis Obispo, CA: Impact Publishers, 1995.

Now try Practice #6.

Practice #6

Assertive Responses:
How to Remain Centered

Instructions. Write assertive responses to the following situations. Practice them to yourself, then practice using these responses when confronted by the situations:

A neighbor is playing music too loud.

Your assertive response: _____

_____

_____

_____

You're taking a friend to a meeting, but the friend keeps puttering around for a half-hour so that you'll arrive late.

Your assertive response: _____

_____

_____

_____

After you've changed to a healthy diet, a friend of yours offers you candy or cookies.

Your assertive response: _____

_____

_____

_____

After you've quit using drugs, an old friend sees you and tries to get you to use, saying, "C'mon, just a little won't hurt. I have some right here."

Your assertive response: _____

_____

_____

_____

What other situation can you think of?

Situation: _____

_____

_____

_____

Your assertive response: _____

_____

_____

_____

Remember, assertiveness is another way to reduce your stress, and clearly, the less stressed you feel, the less you'll want to use drugs.

STRESS MANAGEMENT AND COPING TECHNIQUES

You have just learned how exercise, relaxation techniques, and assertiveness skills can help reduce stress. Here are 22 other effective techniques. Most of them are simple mental exercises anyone can use with a little practice.

Checklist #4

22 Surefire Stress Reducers

Instructions. Go over the list and get a feel for the various coping skills. Which do you like the most? Choose seven or more of these alternatives—the ones you think would work for you. Then, whenever you feel stressed, do one or more of the techniques you have selected.

☐ Imagine a pleasant moment: Maybe you concentrate too much on what goes wrong in your life. Now concentrate on what has gone right. Think of at least one pleasant moment that you experienced in the past week. What were your feelings? How did it happen? Re-create the moment in your mind as fully as you can. Remember it. Dwell on it. Enjoy the utter happiness of that moment once again.

☐ Desensitize stressful moments: If you do concentrate too much on what goes wrong, take a closer look now at what goes wrong. Usually, the trouble isn't so much what has happened as your reaction to it. Visualize something that has gone wrong for you. What was it? Now visualize yourself responding in a positive way to the same situation. Imagine yourself making this positive response the next time the situation arises. Imagine this positive outcome over and over for 10 to 15 minutes. You'll be surprised how much better you'll feel about the situation and how much better you'll deal with the same situation in the future.

☐ Live in the moment: Instead of remembering a pleasant moment from the past, create a pleasant moment now. Live it fully. Concentrate all your attention on a beautiful object, such as a flower or a candle flame. Drop all your thoughts. Don't try to label or describe the beauty—simply experience it in silence. Allow the pleasant sensations to wash over you, and become one with the object of your attention.

☐ Transcendental meditation: Silently or out loud, repeat to yourself a sound, a word, or a phrase, over and over, in rhythmic cadence, for 15 to 20 minutes. Some sounds you can use are "Om," "Aum," "Hum," or "Mmmm." Some words you can use are "One," "God," "Love," or "Sun." Some phrases you can use are "Peace on Earth," "All Is One," "On and On," or "World Without End." It helps if you synchronize the sound with your breathing. Why does this practice work? It helps you focus your mind and become centered.

☐ Silent meditation: Sit comfortably, preferably in a yoga sitting position. Now focus on your breath. Consider this: Your breath is your entire life. Oxygen is food. Without oxygen from breathing, you would die. As you breathe, imagine yourself taking nourishment into all the cells of your body. Breathe deeply and slowly, paying attention to each breath. Gradually, you'll feel the life you gain from breathing and with it a deep sense of gratitude.

☐ Take a vacation: Get away from it all. Go to the shore, the mountains, or anywhere, as long as it offers you a fresh environment. Best bet: Plan a vacation at a health spa and revitalize yourself while you enjoy the new surroundings.

☐ Read a book: Pick your favorite kind of reading material, then kick back and get into it. Kill two birds with one stone? Read a self-help book on how to reduce stress.

☐ Leave work at work: Don't bring work home with you. Don't think about work once you're at home. It's fine to put in extra hours if it doesn't stress you out, but remember to cut back as soon as you feel strain, tension, or fatigue. Look at it this way: If you work eight hours a day and sleep eight hours a day, that leaves you eight hours to yourself. Use them for yourself. Plan leisure activities you like to do—then do them.

☐ Solve problems: If something's bothering you, it's important to identify the problem. Take time to understand the problem—view it from all sides—then solve it. You can solve your own problems or solve any kind of problems you choose. Some people find it relaxing to discover the solutions to various kinds of puzzles and math problems.

☐ Play with a pet: Research shows that playing with a pet lowers blood pressure and heart rate. In other words, it relaxes you. Even more interesting, your pet doesn't have to be a "pettable" pet. Watching fish in an aquarium has been shown to have the same soothing effects.

☐ Sing: Singing is one of the most calming things you can do. When happy, you can sing for joy. When sad, you can sing the blues. Singing expresses feeling. By singing, you let your feelings out, releasing your emotions to the world. So whether it's with a group of friends or in the shower stall, belt out a tune and light up your life with song.

☐ Enjoy plants: Plants bring peaceful feelings. From indoor potted varieties to flower beds to outdoor vegetable gardens, working with plants can be most relaxing. Just looking at plants—or having plants near you—brings a feeling of calm. Extra benefits: Indoor plants brighten your home and freshen the air, flower beds and shrubs beautify your grounds, and vegetable gardens offer peaceful food for a peaceful table. So tend a garden, pot a plant, sow a seed, or prune a bush.

☐ Get into cooking: It's not for everyone, but many people can get totally involved in cooking. Creating a meal can be pleasurable and extremely relaxing. If you're one who can let your cares float away in the kitchen, go for it—bake, broil, chop, sauté, or stir-fry away.

☐ Bathe yourself: Treat yourself to a long, relaxing bath. In soothing, warm to hot water, cares dissolve and tension melts away. Before entering the peaceful waters of your tub, close the bathroom door, lock it, and close your mind to everything outside the room. If you like, add some herbal essence or special fragrance to enhance the effect.

☐ Take a class on stress management: Here's a good way to learn more about reducing your stress. You'll gain many pointers not covered in this book, and in the group you can share your experiences with others.

☐ Walk away: A simple technique: When frustrated with something or someone, walk away. Don't return until you cool down.

- [ ] Do nothing: This option is more like meditation. Do nothing—absolutely nothing. Look at a blank wall. Keep your mind blank. Don't allow a single thought to form. Fight every thought as if it were an intrusion into your imperturbable silence. Do this for 15 to 20 minutes, and you'll feel incredibly refreshed.

- [ ] Groan: Sound peculiar? Well it's not. Groaning helps our bodies handle pain. When you hurt yourself physically—even just stubbing your toe—notice how groaning relieves some of the pain. Groan for a few minutes right now. Notice how it reduces tension. Try it when you want to relax.

- [ ] Cry: This is the ultimate stress reducer. Since the beginning of time, crying has helped the body get rid of inner toxins and release emotional pain. It's the natural response to stress and suffering. Cry whenever you feel the need.

- [ ] Talk it out: If some other person is bothering you, talk it out. Work together with that person to find a common solution. If you can't work with that person to find a solution, talk with someone else. Talking about your problems gets them out in the open and relieves you of most of the stress.

- [ ] Get lost in a fun activity: When disturbed by outside stress, do some activity that you love to do. Dive into your favorite, most fun-filled pastime. Dissolve tension with excitement, gaiety, and amusement.

- [ ] Be thankful: Show gratitude for anything. Gratitude is the most calming emotion there is. Take time to feel thoroughly thankful for a meal, a friend, a family member, your own health, or your ability to change something in your life. Be thankful for life itself.

FRIENDSHIP

*Friendship is a strong and habitual inclination
in two persons to promote the good and
happiness of one another.*
                              —*Eustace Budgell*

There's hardly anything in this world more precious than a friend. A friend can listen to your troubles and help you solve them. Or, if you cannot solve your troubles, a friend will help you feel at peace.

Friendship helps you feel strong inside. Even when everything around you seems gloomy, friendship feels warm. Friendship feels solid. It's one of life's primary needs to know that someone cares for you.

What is a friend? Someone you feel comfortable with. Someone you can tell anything—and everything—about yourself.

Good friends are truthful. They won't lie to you. Perhaps more important, good friends won't let you lie to them.

With a friend, you can talk about your miseries or your shattered dreams, and as you talk, these problems simply drift away. Anger becomes sympathy, resentment turns to forgiveness, and fear converts to love when talking to a friend. Indeed, your best therapist is a good friend.

Practice #7

Find One Good Friend

Instructions. Because friendship is so important to your emotional strength, be sure to have at least one good friend when you quit using drugs. Also be sure that this friend doesn't have a problem with drugs or alcohol.

Most moderate to heavy drug users have two sets of friends, one set that uses and one that doesn't. When you quit the drug use, hang out with your nonusing friends. Choose your best friend from that group and begin seeing that person more often.

Why is this so important? Active drug users normally associate with other users, and they support each other with reasons why they need to keep using. Misery loves company.

However, abruptly changing friends often causes its own problems. That's why it's best to take your time with it. New friends will soon appear. Just keep working toward strong, positive friendships and don't let old, negative friendships drag you down. Remain steadfast and open with everyone.

Who is your best friend? Sometimes the person who you think is your best friend really is not. When you choose a friend, make sure that you can answer yes to all these questions:

> Can I talk confidentially about anything and every-thing with this person?
>
> Can this person help me understand my feelings with-out persuading me to act in a certain way?
>
> Will this person help me make my own decisions?
>
> Do I feel that this person is on my side?
>
> Can we laugh at things together?
>
> Do we enjoy each other's company?
>
> Do I feel that this friendship will endure through time, through difficult periods as well as good periods?

Keep in mind that a lover can be a best friend. If you can't find a best friend among the friends you have, you might find a best friend in your lover—if he or she meets the above criteria.

However, if you can't find anyone at this time to be your best friend, get a therapist. Make sure that you can answer yes to all the above questions when evaluating your therapist as well. Keep looking until you find the therapist who's right for you.

Now, to complete this worksheet, list one person who will be your best friend. Write his or her name here:

_____

If you have a backup best friend (or therapist), write that person's name here:

_____

Of course, be sure to rely on your best friend or backup whenever you feel in need of emotional support.

CHAPTER 9

30 Additional Ways to Renew Yourself

The art of life lies in a constant readjustment to our surroundings.

—*Okarkura Kakuzo*

Using all that you've learned so far, imagine that you were cooking up a cure for drug addiction. Diet would be the main ingredient. Then you would add exercise and relaxation techniques and assertiveness, coping, and friendship skills. Now—just before stirring—it's time to add some spices to make the dish complete.

In this chapter, you'll find the spices: 30 effective methods of healing. Used liberally with the main ingredients, these methods will help cure you of the problems caused by drugs. They will help to heal your body, build your emotional strength, and relax you.

So add some zest to your life. Add some zip. Plan to use at least five or six of these methods in your program for quitting the drugs. You'll have more control over your life and be assured of greater success.

After you read about these methods and consider which ones you would like to do, you can select the ones you will do in Worksheet #7.

ACUPUNCTURE

This relatively new method for treating drug addiction and alcoholism increases success rates with many individuals. It just might work for you.

Actually, acupuncture is not new. Refined and cultivated for about 3,000 years in the Far East, this proven method has finally gained widespread acceptance in the United States.

What is acupuncture? It involves rechanneling the energy of the body for the purpose of healing. You can receive treatments for almost any kind of ailment, including simple pain. The treatment for drug and alcohol addiction involves inserting five very thin, short needles into points on the outer ear for 30 to 45 minutes. This treatment is so easy that it can be done in a waiting room on a walk-in basis.

How does acupuncture work? Stimulating these points on the outer ear creates an energy exchange with the brain, causing it to automatically produce endorphins. Instantly, you experience a natural high—with no drugs and no alcohol. Thus, not only is the treatment completely painless, but it generates feelings of total euphoria. Eighty percent of individuals receiving this treatment report an improvement in how they feel. (Among the remaining 20%, it should be noted that some of them felt some pain from the needles.)

Current studies on acupuncture show that this method can help during the withdrawal and early recovery from cocaine, heroin, or alcohol. Ideally, long-term results would show a decrease in the need for acupuncture treatment as the brain regained control of its own endorphin production.

Check your area for acupuncture clinics or holistic health centers. Also consult drug and alcohol treatment centers. Many now offer acupuncture on an out-patient basis.

Acupressure. Acupressure attempts to achieve the same results as acupuncture without the needles by applying pressure through finger massage and squeezing. It's an effective treatment, but not as powerful as acupuncture. You might prefer an acupressure massage, called shiatsu, to relax the whole body. (For information on acupressure and massage, see the next section.)

Another Variation: CES. CES stands for Cranial Electrostimulation (also known as NET, which is short for neuroelectric therapy). For this treatment, adhesive electrodes are attached to ear points (behind the ear so as not to be too visible), and wires connect to a stimulator worn on a belt or put in a pocket. It uses a button that can send a mild current to the ear points. This current causes stimulation—similar to the effects of acupuncture—that prompts the brain to produce endorphins. The interesting plus about CES is that you can get the stimulation anytime you need it. If you feel a little down, just press a button.

For specific information on CES/NET, read the book *Hooked? NET: The New Approach to Drug Cure*, by Meg Patterson, M.B.E., M.B.Ch.B., F.R.C.S.E. (London: Faber and Faber, 1986). To get your own CES machine, contact Tools for Exploration in San Raphael, California. For their catalog, call 888-748-6657.

MASSAGE

When you bang into something and hurt yourself, what's the first thing you do? Rub the sore spot—and for good reason. Rubbing soothes the area and diminishes the pain.

A massage is nothing more than a good rub—to soothe the entire body. It helps reduce tension, release stress, and dissolve your aches and pains. In addition, many professionals claim a great amount of healing power for various types of massage.

It's one thing to exchange massages with loved ones or friends—you might want to do that—but also be sure to try a few sessions with one or more local professionals. You'll be amazed at the incredible transformation that you can achieve at the hands of a professional.

When seeking a professional massage, you might find the following descriptions of types of massage helpful:

Acupressure/Shiatsu. Based on the acupuncture medical model for improving energy flow in the body, this involves deep pressing with the fingers, knuckles, and thumbs. It's warming. It increases circulation, relieves tension, and improves the healing of internal organs.

Swedish Massage. Softer than acupressure, this method is characterized by long, smooth strokes, usually with the open hand. Relaxing and warming, it releases tension in muscles.

Sports Massage. This more active kind of rubbing with the open hand involves some percussion, or drumming, on the body with the hands. It's good for releasing muscle tension, including muscle cramps, and for increasing circulation.

Rolfing. Perhaps the most intense and comprehensive of all massages (10 sessions to complete the course), this method, named for its inventor, Ida Rolf, involves everything from soft, smooth touch to hard, almost painful kneading of deep tissue. It is said to "realign" the body, balance the mind, correct internal energies, and heal bodily organs. Many prominent people have been Rolfed and give glowing testimonials.

For more information on various alternatives, call Associated Bodywork and Massage Professionals (Evergreen, Colorado) at 303-674-8478 or American Massage Therapy Association (Evanston, Illinois) at 847-864-0123.

BIOFEEDBACK

When you feel good, your brain produces alpha waves. Exercise, meditation, restful sleep, and creative activity all stimulate the production of alpha waves. When the alpha waves flow, your mind is relaxed.

The original biofeedback machines measured alpha waves, and when the brain emitted a certain level of alpha, the machine gave a signal. By this process people learned how to increase their own alpha output. More important, once they had learned it and practiced it, they didn't need the equipment anymore. They could go into "alpha state" at will, almost any time of the day, whenever they needed to relax.

Now biofeedback machines can help you control many of the so-called involuntary bodily functions. For example, you can learn to raise or lower your heart rate at will. You can learn to reduce muscle tension, body temperature, and nervousness. All these learned responses are surefire ways to reduce stress and increase your feelings of relaxation.

To get yourself connected to a biofeedback machine, try your local mental health clinic or a psychotherapist.

To buy your own, contact Tools for Exploration at 888-748-6657.

BODYWORK/BODY MOVEMENT

You have studied many forms of bodywork already: various exercises, yoga, stretching, and so on. A list of some additional forms follows. Each can help heal you and reduce your stress.

Tai Chi. A beautiful form of bodily motion with exercises based on energy balancing, it's said to have internal healing power.

Martial Arts. Tae kwan do, kung fu, karate, jujitsu, akido. Exercises facilitate strength, coordination, and movement.

Alexander Technique. This involves methods for body balancing and working with spinal alignment in your normal everyday activity.

Feldenkrais Method. A series of "body lessons" that increase your awareness of inner movement, flexibility, and coordination.

Ohashiatsu. Teaches you to balance internal energies through movements and self-massage.

And many more techniques are available: Rubenfeld synergy, Trager mind-body integration, polarity therapy, and Neo-Reichian/bioenergetics. All these use various combinations of methods to help you balance your energy, heal internal organs, and relax.

These methods work with varying degrees of effectiveness for different individuals. Experiment to find which work best for you.

Where can you find listings of providers of these techniques? Check any "new age" directory in your area as well as alternative newspapers and magazines. If you have a holistic health center nearby, call and ask for information on what it offers.

HYPNOSIS

Through the power of suggestion, a hypnotist can plant a thought in your mind that you'll remember after the session. This can help you in two ways. First, the hypnotist can coax you to feel more relaxed in certain situations that would normally bother you. Second, the hypnotist can create powerful built-in reminders to help you control your desire to use drugs.

Over the past few decades, hypnotists have achieved great success in these two areas. Unfortunately, hypnosis doesn't work for everyone. Only about 50% of the population can be hypnotized, and among those who can, only about 5% to 10% find that it helps them break an addiction.

If you think you're interested in hypnosis, check it out. First see if you are able to be hypnotized, then go from there.

AUTOGENIC TRAINING/SELF-HYPNOSIS

Research shows that individuals can learn to relax by lying comfortably with the eyes closed and repeating certain key phrases to themselves. This is called autogenic training or self-hypnosis. Sample phrases include "My breath is calm and regular," "My heartbeat feels slow and certain," "My body feels heavy," "I feel warm all over," and "My nerves will settle now."

A trained therapist can help you get started, then you can do it on your own. Or you can just start by doing it on your own—it's not that hard. (By the way, autogenic training coupled with biofeedback has been shown to be doubly effective. If you choose one, you might want to choose the other.)

VISUALIZATION

Please take a moment to relax. Now imagine yourself sucking on a lemon. Imagine the tart taste of lemon juice filling your mouth. What does it feel like on your tongue? What does it feel like at the back of your throat when you swallow? Now stop the image and check yourself. Your mouth is slightly puckered and loaded with saliva. Why? Your imagination is so powerful that it can actually change what happens to you physically.

To be sure, whatever you imagine about yourself can dramatically change your life. When you're sick and you imagine yourself healing the ailment, studies show that you have a much better chance of getting well. These studies have documented improved success with a variety of ailments, physical problems, and diseases, including cancer.

How can you use this technique when you quit the drugs? After you quit, visualize yourself getting well. Visualize your body healing the many physical ailments that drugs have caused. Visualize yourself in the image of health.

Imagine a war being waged inside yourself. Imagine yourself winning. Over and over, imagine yourself winning and gaining the reward of good health.

Here's yet another way that visualization can help: Imagine yourself resisting the temptation to use a drug. Imagine yourself saying (inside yourself), "I don't need it anymore. I've outgrown it. I prefer to be healthy now. I want to be free. It's time now for me to grow up." Imagine yourself going through a heroic transformation. Visualize yourself getting better and better.

Visualization can help in another way, too. Imagine yourself in a situation in which someone, maybe an old friend, is coaxing you to use. Imagine yourself refusing. Imagine yourself refusing politely yet firmly. Imagine exactly what you'll say to the person, something like, "No thanks, I've quit for health reasons. This drug has been harming me for too long, and I can't use it anymore." Practice saying your reason over and over.

One other way in which you can practice visualization: Whenever you think about using a drug, imagine your worst high on that drug. Remember it completely. Maybe you nearly died or felt like you could have died. Maybe you embarrassed yourself beyond belief, made a mistake that cost you thousands of dollars (in wrecked automobiles, legal fees, hospital bills, and so on), or seriously hurt someone. Now imagine yourself avoiding these kinds of problems completely. Imagine becoming proud of yourself for doing well in life. Imagine all this as one of your main reasons to avoid the drug.

AFFIRMATIONS

This technique combines some elements of both self-hypnosis and visualization. An affirmation is a positive statement about yourself that you repeat over and over again until your subconscious gets the message. Here's a way to say yes to yourself—a way to change and to help yourself grow.

Here's the technique: Choose your affirmation and repeat it over and over. Repeat it silently to yourself. Repeat it out loud whenever you can. Also write it. Write the entire affirmation over and over, 20 to 30 times at a sitting. Do this at least once a day.

To get you started, here are some ideas for affirmations. You can change the words of any affirmation to make it sound more like you. Select one or two affirmations and keep working with them until you feel yourself changing.

To help with quitting:

My body keeps regaining health.

I am becoming strong.

I envision myself thinking clearly now.

I see myself in control of my thoughts and actions.

I feel comfortable in my body.

I choose not to use drugs.

I will avoid drugs—they have been ruining my life.

I will avoid _____ (name of drug)—it has been ruining my life.

I want to be healthy.

I will find greater happiness.

My body radiates health.

My body radiates happiness.

Now I choose to grow.

Now I will mature.

Now I'm in control.

I am free to be myself.

To handle guilt over past actions:

> I forgive myself for mistakes I've made.
>
> I forgive myself for hurting myself.
>
> I can't change the past. It's done and gone. But I will change the future.

From Sondra Ray's book *Loving Relationships:*

> I forgive myself for hurting others.
>
> I forgive myself for struggling in life.
>
> I forgive others for hurting me.
>
> I am innocent. I am a child of God. All my desires are holy and they always have been.

You can find many other affirmations—and ways to use them—in Ray's book, which I recommend.

SUBLIMINAL SUGGESTION

Today, various audio- and videotapes are available that make use of subliminal suggestion. These tapes promise to help you change something about yourself. Some of the subjects include how to break a drug addiction, how to quit drinking, how to quit smoking, and how to relax.

How do they work? The audiotapes have a soundtrack of music or ocean waves and a secondary, inaudible soundtrack that is nevertheless perceived by your subconscious mind. The videotapes present some pleasant visual scene with visual messages interspersed at $\frac{1}{46}$th of a second—too fast for your eye to see yet perceptible to your subconscious. At the same time, the video's soundtrack is embedded with subliminal vocal messages.

These messages are much like the affirmations just described. Here's a sampling of messages from two different subliminal tapes on quitting drugs:

I can say "No Drugs."

I just say "NO!"

I am in control.

I like myself.

(From "Say No to Drugs and Say Yes to a Brighter Future," by Success Education Institute International, San Diego, CA; phone: 800-248-2737).

I feel good on my own.

I can handle my life naturally.

I am relaxed and calm about substances.

I am feeling great.

(From "Stop Drug Abuse," by Tools for Exploration, San Raphael, CA; phone: 888-748-6657).

You can find other tapes with other variations. But, when you select a subliminal tape, make sure that its messages match your feelings. For example, if you don't like the phrase "I just say NO!", the first tape mentioned above will not work well for you.

Subliminal tapes don't work for everyone. In fact, when measured scientifically, visualization and affirmation techniques show higher success rates. However, you might want to try all three of these methods to see what works best for you.

A CLINIC OR A LIVE-IN PROGRAM

Ever think of taking some time off and going somewhere for intensive treatment? It might be just what you need. The right treatment center, clinic, or health resort can greatly improve your chances for success.

Why? Because it gives you an opportunity to reorganize yourself in a safe environment. At your own pace, you can change your ways. Moreover, getting away from the environment you associate with your habits and problems and away from the daily struggle of coping can do wonders.

Does this sound like it could be for you? If so, plan to go to a clinic or enter a live-in program soon after you have quit the drugs. Probably the best time for this is immediately after detoxification. In fact, many treatment facilities combine detox with an ongoing program. The detox phase might take four to seven days, and a live-in phase might take another seven to 25 days or more. Also, the clinic might keep you on an outpatient basis for as long as a year or perhaps longer.

Many different types of clinics and live-in programs, offering a wide variety of services, are available. Also, keep in mind that most treatment programs are covered by medical insurance.

What kind of services can you expect?

Most drug and alcohol treatment centers and clinics base their approach on the so-called Minnesota model developed in Hazelden in the 1950s. These centers offer mainly three things: psychotherapy, education, and the 12-Step programs of AA and NA. Studies at these centers have shown that their three-year success rates are fairly low (between 5% and 25%).

However, a new kind of center, started in the 1980s, offers a broader approach to recovery, called the whole-person approach. These centers treat all aspects of the individual: the physical, the emotional, the mental, and the spiritual. The key addition here is the physical. These new centers address physical healing and biochemical repair of the individual. Techniques include nutritional therapy, dietary counseling, exercise, stress reduction techniques, and relaxation skills.

Of course, when individuals can reduce their physical stress, they can achieve greater healing mentally, emotionally, and spiritually as well. This overall healing shows in the success rates of centers offering a whole-person approach. Studies reveal that one-, two-, and three-year success rates for these centers range from 50% to 90%.

Among these centers, most still incorporate AA or NA as part of their overall programs. In fact, some require that you attend AA or NA, yet other centers make it optional, and some have dropped AA and NA altogether. However, whether or not AA or NA is included, look for a center that offers a whole-person approach to recovery. This center should have a strong component for physical healing, including stress reduction, exercise, and relaxation techniques, and a plan for dietary intervention as well.

To help break a heroin addiction, you might prefer the long-term-withdrawal method offered at a methadone or LAAM clinic. At one of these, you trade your heroin addiction for methadone or LAAM. Then, over the course of a few months to a year or more, you gradually wean yourself from the methadone or LAAM.

Of course, for healing purposes, don't feel limited to drug rehabilitation centers. You can find many different kinds of health resorts and spiritual retreats across the country. Once you complete detox, you can choose any of these that suit you.

The July/August 1998 issue of the magazine *Healing Retreats & Spas* lists, by state, about 920 wellness centers in its "National Retreat, Spa, and Yoga Directory." Of course, the 12-Step philosophy will be of little concern at these centers, but the programs they offer can help renew you.

SOLITUDE AND SELF-REFLECTION

How do you feel about being alone? Perhaps you like it. Perhaps you find that you gain strength whenever you take an hour or two to be completely by yourself.

If so, you have plenty of company. Many people need to make time for themselves, away from the crowd, to sort things out alone.

Solitude is one of life's most rewarding experiences. It gives you a chance to examine yourself and make plans for self-renewal. It can be a time for artistic creation, self-reflection, resolution, or inner peace.

Use your solitude to your advantage, and it can revitalize you.

A precaution: You must be relaxed. If you spend your time alone, nervously worrying about yourself, it will do no good. Best bet: If you feel nervous or anxious, take care of that first. Then your solitude will be calming, and your self-reflection will bring strength.

For over 300 quotations on the nature, importance, and power of solitude, read *The Wonders of Solitude* (Dale Salwak, ed. Novato, CA: New World Library, 1998).

HEALING WITH LAUGHTER

Ho, ho, ho, ha, ha, hee, hee, hee. Laugh right now. Notice how it calms you? A hearty laugh not only calms the body but also helps it to heal.

Studies show that laughter, like exercise, produces endorphins, the body's natural tranquilizers. Other studies show that laughter stimulates the immune system by increasing antibodies and lowering cortisol. That means laughter promotes physical healing and greater strength against disease.

So laugh it up. Enjoy something funny. Give a great guffaw. Chuckle, bellow, ha ha ha. Here are some suggestions:

Watch comedians or a funny movie on television.

Go to comedy clubs.

Read the comics.

Hang around funny people: jokesters, pranksters, and so on.

Go to a circus to see the clowns (or hire a clown to come to your home for birthday parties).

Read a funny book: a joke book or a humorous novel.

Look for more humor in yourself, in every little thing you do.

Act silly; clown around whenever you can.

Look for more humor in the universe. Meditate on this. Our universe is really a very funny place, you know.

TURN OFF YOUR TELEVISION

Television increases your nervous energy in two ways. First, it keeps you inactive, sitting in front of the set. Second, it blasts your body with a constant barrage of electrons.

How does television work? An electron gun shoots electrons at the screen. This produces the image. But the electrons don't stop at the screen. They come right through the screen and enter the human body. This "electron bath" can be very dangerous. Electrons, which are negatively charged electrical particles, can wreak havoc on your nervous system. Why? Your nervous system depends on a balance of positive and negative charges.

Laboratory rats placed in front of a color television showed extreme hyperactivity for the first 10 days to a month. Their behavior during this time was nervous, restless, and even aggressive and hostile. Then the animals began to show fatigue. They became so lethargic that they needed a push just to get them to move around the cage. Other studies have found that if two color televisions sets are aimed at young rats, many of them die. The reason? Autopsies indicated severe brain tissue damage.

Not only does television make you nervous and interfere with mental functioning, it takes precious time that you could be using to do something positive for yourself. For example, you could be exercising— something that actually reduces depression and fatigue. You could be reading an important book, taking a night class, building something, creating something, or having fun.

Now let's back up for a minute. Some television shows may be exceptions. You might actually gain some benefits from the following:

Watching educational programming that can help you learn something important.

Watching exercise programs (or exercise video-tapes) *while doing the exercises.*

Watching a show that makes you laugh—for example, a comedy routine or some really hilarious show. A sitcom that forces you to sit through a half-hour of drudgery for two or three laughs isn't worth it.

So what to do? Cut out almost all television. Allow yourself eight to 10 hours a week, maximum. This includes anything that you watch on videotape as well.

The less television, the better. How will you do it? Plan your week ahead of time. For example, you might want to watch three or four shows during the week and a movie or sporting event on the weekend. Make up your mind. If this is your plan, stick to it—don't watch any more television that week.

FASTING

Here's a healing method as old as the human race itself. Also, animals use it regularly. When sick, animals will naturally stop eating for a while until they get better. Humans have the same instinct. In all cultures, throughout history, we have used fasting as a primary method of healing.

But fasting does more than just heal the body. It can clear your thoughts and illuminate your mind. All of the world's greatest spiritual leaders have used fasting as a means to inner enlightenment—Jesus, Buddha, Muhammad, Gandhi, to name just a few.

How does fasting help? It rids the body of toxins, leading the way to better health. The body routinely stores toxins and unwanted chemical buildup in body fat. A fast breaks down the body fat, thereby releasing the toxins into the bloodstream. The body then excretes the toxins through normal channels of elimination.

There are many kinds of fasts and methods of fasting. Here's a brief overview:

> Normal daily fasting. Go about 12 hours without food every day, say, from 7:00 in the evening until 7:00 the next morning. This gives the body time to get rid of some unwanted chemical buildup and metabolic debris. You break your fast with breakfast.

Only two meals a day. One at 3:00 PM and one at 7:00 PM This kind of fast gives the body an even longer break.

One or two full days (or more). This can help clear the body of a great amount of excess junk. After a full two days, you begin to get into spiritual fasting. However, if you plan to go more than two days, it's best to get supervision. Many health resorts offer supervised fasting.

Water fast. You need to drink lots of liquids on a fast. If you're a purist, you might drink only water.

Juice fast. The liquid of choice: fresh squeezed natural organic juices. This is probably the best liquid for fasting because the alkalizing effects of the juice offset the acid-forming effects of toxins being released into the bloodstream. Vegetable broth can also be used with just about the same effects as juice.

(Note: *Do not* attempt to fast if you are more than 10 pounds underweight, if you have any serious illness, if you are pregnant, or if you are a lactating mother.)

By the way, fasting specifically helps to cure addictions. Why? Because addictions leave incredible amounts of toxic buildup in the body. Gabriel Cousins, doctor of medicine and dietary counselor, in his column in the September 1989 issue of *New Frontier Magazine,* said that fasting is "excellent for helping addictions to food, cigarettes, and other drugs. When toxins are removed (by fasting), the cell memory of that to which one was addicted is changed. That is why the body tends to resist junk, polluted or artificial food, and drugs after a fast."

Before choosing to fast, get more details. Learn as much as you can. Talk to a holistic dietary counselor or read more about it. Two books that can help are Annemarie Colbin's *Food and Healing* and Carrie L'Esperance's *The Ancient Cookfire: How to Rejuvenate Body and Spirit Through Seasonal Foods and Fasting.*

INTESTINAL CLEANSING

If you've been a moderate to heavy drug user, chances are that you have some kind of bowel trouble. You might have irritable bowel syndrome, colitis, Crohn's disease, or chronic constipation.

The best ongoing treatment for these is a good diet (as outlined in Chapter 6). However, you might also benefit from colonic cleansing.

For starters, colonic cleansing solves one very serious problem: It removes built-up fecal matter that has lodged in the intestines over the course of years. Some people have up to five pounds of accumulated waste stuck to the lining of their intestines. Researchers associate the greatest fecal accumulations with diets high in fat, especially animal fat (meat, eggs, milk, butter, cheese, yogurt, and ice cream). Needless to say, this backlog of bodily waste impedes the normal functioning of the intestines and causes disease.

On the other hand, a colonic or an enema can remove this buildup and give you a fresh start. No doubt, you'll view this as good news. However, keep in mind that colonics and enemas should not be done too often.

Use a colonic maybe once a year, and consider it only if you've been eating poorly. An enema can be used occasionally to help with constipation. However, if used too often, you can become dependent on it as easily as you can become dependent on laxatives.

If you choose this option, you might want to do it for yourself, or you might want to have it administered professionally. You can find many health resorts and holistic healing centers offering this service. Just check around.

HERBAL REMEDIES

Many plants and herbs have the power to heal. Ever since the dawn of civilization, these have been studied and classified. Indeed, for thousands of years these natural cures were the only medicines known.

Now, in the modern day, you can find herbal remedies for nearly any kind of complaint. Entire books have been devoted to the subject. You might want to use one of the following books as a guide: *The Way of Herbs*, by Michael Tierra, C.A., N.D. (New York: Washington Square Press, 1980) or *Medicine of the Earth*, by Susanne Fischer-Rizzi (Portland, OR: Rudra Press, 1996). In addition, you might also want to get advice from a naturopathic doctor (N.D.) or other holistic health professional.

Meanwhile, to give you an idea, here are two lists of herbal health remedies: one for stress reduction and one to promote general physical healing.

Stress Reducers

Chamomile: Relaxant; reduces anxiety, induces sleep

Lady's slipper: Reduces anxiety, lifts mood, helps cure depression

Passionflower: Sedative, induces sleep

St. John's wort: Reduces anxiety, tension, and fatigue

Scullcap: Sedative; lifts depression, revitalizes nervous system

Valerian: Sedative; reduces tension

Vervain: Sedative; relieves depression and sadness

Wood betony: Relaxant, sedative; eases nervousness, relieves headaches due to nervousness

Internal Healers

Chaparral: Antiseptic, antibiotic; stimulates the immune system

Echinacea: Antibiotic; good for acute infections, regulates white blood cell count

Garlic: Antibiotic; increases the body's resistance to infection

Ginseng: Strengthens the immune system, increases resistance to stress, builds stamina, renews sexual vitality

Goldenseal: Fights bacteria, helps cure infections (especially of throat and chest)

Marigold: Stimulates white blood cell and interferon production

Pau d'arco: Anti-yeast, antifungal agent

Peppermint: Good for stomachache, stimulates internal cleansing, strengthens the body

Thyme: Stimulates internal cleansing, strengthens the body

One caution: These herbs are very powerful. A little, once in a while, might be good for you, but too much can harm you. Use them only as needed, until you experience the healing benefits, and then stop. Herbs can be taken with water or made into a mild tea and sipped.

AROMATHERAPY

For thousands of years, scents and fragrances have been used for healing and mood-changing purposes. Consider the mood created by incense burning at a spiritual service or the power of various perfumes and body lotions to stimulate sexual desire. Consider a fragrant potpourri that blithely lifts your mood or the scent of a certain bath oil that totally relaxes you.

Aromatherapy is a form of herbal healing. You use various plants and herbs that impart active ingredients in their scents or aromas. By simply smelling or inhaling the active ingredients, you can experience a physical change inside.

You can find aroma cures for many kinds of ailments. Here are a few that are recommended to alleviate depression and nervousness:

Almond oil: Relaxant; reduces nervousness

Chamomile: Mood lifter, relaxant

Lavender: Relaxant

Lemon oil: Mood lifter; reduces depression

Melissa: Relaxant

Narcissus: Relaxant

Peppermint: Mood lifter; reduces depression

Pine oil: Mood lifter

Rose: Mood lifter, calmative; reduces depression

Sandalwood: Relaxant

Spearmint: Mood lifter

Ylang-ylang: Relaxant

For best results, use the pure essential oils from these natural products. The oils can be simply smelled from the bottle, misted into the air, added to a hot bath, or gently massaged into your skin.

For more information on fragrances and many useful therapies, see *Essential Aromatherapy,* by Susan Worwood (San Raphael, CA: New World Library, 1995).

HOMEOPATHY

A complete health care system in itself, homeopathy uses plant, mineral, and animal substances to stimulate healing. You can use this system not only to cure common ailments but also to improve your general long-term health and well-being.

You won't find a specific cure for drug addiction, but you can use homeopathy to heal many of the ailments caused by drug addiction.

For additional information, see *Everybody's Guide to Homeopathic Medicine* (Cummings, Stephen, with Dana Ullman, M.P.H. New York: Putnam Group–Jeremy P. Tarcher [revised edition], 1997) or go to a homeopathic professional for specific remedies and advice.

CHIROPRACTIC

What comes to your mind when you think of chiropractic? Works well for back problems, right? Well, chiropractic isn't just for back problems.

As you probably know, the spinal cord carries the main energy flow inside your body. By aligning spinal vertebrae, chiropractors enhance this energy flow, increasing "communication" through the spinal cord and all the peripheral nerves. In turn, this process reduces stress and promotes inner healing as the nerve networks and pathways are unblocked and resensitized.

Chiropractic offers one of the best methods of regaining health for the drug user whose nerves have been numbed by years of using.

Check for a chiropractor or chiropractic clinic near you.

A CHEMICAL DETERRENT TO DRUG USE

If drugs stopped bringing pleasurable effects, you would probably stop using, right? If you're an opiate user, you can actually make this happen. There is a drug, naltrexone, that blocks the effects of opiates.

Some heroin addicts have been able to use naltrexone successfully to help them break the habit. However, studies show that the overall percentage of addicts who have been successful with the drug is low.

Nevertheless, it might be for you. It might give you that extra boost, that extra feeling of self-control that you need. Perhaps you can stop taking the naltrexone after six months to a year, or whenever you feel your willpower is strong enough to keep you away from the opiates. Naltrexone won't be any problem to walk away from because it's nonaddicting.

If you want to start on naltrexone, go to a medical doctor. You need to take it under supervision—and you need a prescription.

ALTERNATIVE APPROACHES TO QUITTING DRUGS

You already know about the 12-Step approach. This approach has dominated formal addiction treatment since the 1950s. Of course, most people who have quit serious addictions have done so informally, without the ongoing use of any treatment program. As evidence of this, a scientific Gallup poll reported recently, "People are about 10 times more likely to change on their own as with the help of doctors (physicians), therapists, or self-help groups." The survey found that "professional help had surprisingly little to do with important life changes, even health-related ones. Doctors helped people change only 3% of the time, while psychologists and psychiatrists, self-help groups and religious counselors got the credit even less often. Support was much more likely to come from friends (14%), parents, children, or siblings (21%), or a spouse, boyfriend, or girlfriend (29%). And 30% of the time, people simply did what they had to do on their own, often with striking success."

People gain help and support from many different places. What works for you might not work for someone else. That's why it's important to have many avenues to treatment.

In this book, you have one of the new alternatives to the 12-Step program. However, many other programs are currently available to you. Some of these are "group programs," programs that offer a national network of groups that, like AA and NA, meet in a regular place on a regular basis. And some of these are "individual programs," programs that individuals can use on their own.

Six Group Programs

You can call or write to any of the following groups for more information or to find a meeting near you:

Women for Sobriety (WFS)
P.O. Box 618
Quakertown, PA 18951
215-536-8026; 800-333-1606

Founder: Jean Kirkpatrick, Ph.D.
Started: 1975
Number of groups in U.S.: 200 to 250
Growth outside the U.S.: Many groups have been started in Finland, Ireland, and Australia.

Background: When Jean Kirkpatrick had quit her alcoholic drinking, she found that AA didn't work for her. One reason: In mixed groups such as AA, men tend to dominate discussion, and this often leaves women feeling intimidated or frustrated. Yet, what women need most in recovery is to build self-esteem.

So, WFS offers Thirteen Statements of Acceptance to help people live a life free of alcohol and drugs. In contrast to the 12 steps, these statements are nonreligious thoughts that help members become more self-reliant in everyday life and achieve a lasting and successful recovery.

Also, WFS incorporates a whole-person approach. As part of its program, WFS gives recommendations to help with physical healing, including a dietary plan and guidelines for exercise.

See the following books by Jean Kirkpatrick about the program: *Goodbye Hangovers, Hello Life: Self-Help for Women* (Quakertown, PA: WFS, 1996) and *Turnabout: New Help for the Woman Alcoholic* (New York: Bantam, 1990).

Men for Sobriety (MFS)

P.O. Box 618
Quakertown, PA 18951
215-536-8026; 800-333-1606

Founder: Jean Kirkpatrick, Ph.D.
Started: 1990
Number of members active in groups: 100
Number of groups in U.S.: 10

Background: The WFS program works for men, too. Indeed, the program's basic concepts apply to both men and women. For example, men find that the Thirteen Statements of Acceptance are strong esteem builders and, like women, can use them as helpful building blocks to a successful recovery.

Secular Organizations for Sobriety (SOS); also known as **Save Our Selves**
5521 Grosvenor Blvd.
Los Angeles, CA 90066
310-821-8430

Founder: James Christopher
Started: 1986
Number of groups in U.S.: 1,100 (about 700 of these operate in prisons and halfway houses in Texas, where inmates can choose SOS as an alternative to the AA or NA groups that are also available.

Growth outside the U.S.: This program had a major growth spurt in foreign membership (in the early 1990s) through an alliance with secular recovery groups in Europe. It has a strong presence in France, Poland, the Netherlands, and Australia.

Background: When Jim Christopher had quit his alcoholic drinking, he tried AA, only to find that it didn't work for him. The main problem was the religiosity of the Twelve Step program. So, he started SOS as a secular alternative for people who need to break alcohol and drug addictions.

Instead of 12 steps, SOS offers six Suggested Guidelines for Sobriety. These powerful ideas are designed to help you take control of your life.

Two keys to SOS: First, every day you acknowledge that sobriety is your "Number 1" priority. This is called your Sobriety Priority. Second, you keep your own personal Journal of Recovery, a specifically designed workbook covering 52 weeks of the year. In SOS as well as other programs, the journal technique has proven an extremely successful adjunct to recovery.

See the following books by James Christopher about the program: *Unhooked: Staying Sober and Drug-Free* (Buffalo, NY: Prometheus Books, 1989) and *SOS Sobriety: The Proven Alternative to 12 Step Programs* (Buffalo, NY: Prometheus Books, 1992).

Rational Recovery (RR)
Box 800
Lotus, CA 95651
530-621-4374; 800-303-CURE

Founder: Jack Trimpey, L.C.S.W.
Started: 1986
Number of groups in U.S.: 200 to 300
Background: When Jack Trimpey tried to break his addiction to alcohol, the 12-Step program didn't work for him. He felt that the moralizing of AA, the required religiosity, and the idea of powerlessness were not helpful to most people and in fact could be detrimental to someone trying to make a constructive change. That's why he developed RR—to provide a "rational alternative."

Based on the Addictive Voice Recognition Technique (AVRT), RR teaches its members to identify the addictive voice within—to recognize the inner voice that keeps urging you to drink or use drugs—and to fight it. The addictive voice represents the irrational side of you called, intimately, "the beast." RR gives you many methods that help you fight the beast and 14 "Rational Ideas" that you can use as guidelines to successful recovery.

RR has another goal: It teaches its members to avoid all types of dependency, including dependency on groups and "regular meetings." So, although RR still has some groups in operation, it attempts to "graduate" its members from these as quickly as possible.

See the following book by Jack Trimpey about the program: *Rational Recovery: The New Cure for Substance Addiction* (New York: Pocket Books, 1996).

Discovery Empowerment Groups (also known as "16-Step Groups")
Box 1302
Lolo, MT 59847
406-273-6068

Founder: Charlotte Davis Kasl, Ph.D.
Started: 1992
Number of groups in U.S.: 100 to 200
Growth outside of the U.S.: A few groups have been started in Canada and Mexico.
Background: Charlotte Kasl developed her "empowerment group" model as an alternative to the traditional 12 step model. She has observed that AA/NA's notion of powerlessness actually engendered helplessness in many people. So in her program, she encourages people to know their choices and learn how to empower themselves to change.

Central to the Discovery Empowerment Groups are Kasl's "16 Steps for Discovery and Empowerment." These steps help individuals with key needs during the recovery process and cover all areas—physical, mental, emotional, and spiritual.

See the following books by Charlotte Kasl about her recovery program and her 16-Step Groups: *Many Roads, One Journey: Moving Beyond the 12 Steps* (New York: Harper Perennial, 1992) and *Yes, You Can! A Guide to Empowerment Groups* (Lolo, MT: Castle Consulting, 1995).

Self-Management and Recovery Training (SMART)
24000 Mercantile Rd., Suite 11
Beachwood, OH 44122
216-292-0220

Founders: Many professionals in the addiction treatment field who organized as the Alcohol and Drug Abuse Self-Help Network, Inc., doing business as Self-Management and Recovery Training (SMART).

Started: 1994

Number of groups in U.S.: 275

Background: A core group of drug and alcohol treatment professionals based this program on the therapeutic intervention known as Rational Emotive Behavioral Therapy (REBT). REBT was developed by Dr. Albert Ellis, and it has a strong track record in the treatment of addictions.

SMART emphasizes four key steps in recovery: (1) enhancing motivation, (2) refusing to act on urges to use, (3) managing life's problems in a sensible and effective way, and (4) developing a positive, balanced, and healthy lifestyle. In the SMART program, you receive many practical "behavioral" techniques (things to do) to help you with all four of these steps. You'll learn how thinking creates feelings and how to change your thinking in a way that helps to change your feelings.

See the following books about SMART recovery (available through SMART headquarters): *Member's Manual* (Beechwood, OH: SMART Recovery, 1996) and *S.M.A.R.T. Recovery: A Sensible Primer* (revised edition), by William Knaus, Ph.D. (Longmeadow, MA: William Knaus, 1998).

Individual Programs

Currently, you can find at least 20 self-help programs that can be used as alternatives to the 12-Step approach.

All of these have been described in books. Here are six of the most notable:

Changing for Good: The Revolutionary Program That Explains the Six Stages of Change and Teaches You How to Free Yourself from Bad Habits, by James Prochaska, Ph.D., John Norcross, Ph.D., and Carlo DiClemente, Ph.D. New York: Morrow, 1994.

Based on 12 years of research and more than 50 studies involving more than $35 million in research funding, this book offers a new paradigm for self-change with a proven high success rate.

Help Yourself: A Revolutionary Alternative Recovery Program, by Dr. Joel C. Robertson. Nashville: Thomas Nelson, 1992.

Dr. Robertson, director of The Robertson Institute, Ltd., in Michigan, specializes in neuropharmacology (brain chemistry technology). His book serves as an in-depth workbook that will help you at all levels: physical, mental, emotional, and spiritual. After you determine your personal nature, you choose techniques to meet your specific needs.

Rational Madness: The Paradox of Addiction, by Ray Hoskins. Blue Ridge Summit, PA: Tab Books, 1989.

This book presents an extremely enlightening view of addictive behavior. When you peel away one layer of addiction (such as alcohol or drug addiction), you find other layers of addiction. These include food addictions, various mental compulsions, and "behavior addictions" such as addictions to work, gambling, sex, and relationships. The book offers techniques, mainly psychological and spiritual, to help you work through these layers of addiction and become free.

The Recovery Book, by Al J. Mooney, M.D., Arlene Eisenberg, and Howard Eisenberg. New York: Workman, 1992.

This giant 600-page guide looks at all aspects of recovery. The 12-Step programs are mentioned often as a recovery technique, but the book also answers hundreds of questions about recovery in non-12-step terms. You'll find that this book serves very much as an encyclopedia, covering the entire recovery field with useful information and state-of-the-art advice.

Recovery from Addiction, by John Finnegan and Daphne Gray. Berkeley, CA: Celestial Arts, 1990.

The authors urge a whole-person approach to recovery and give suggestions to guide the reader. This book presents a strong dietary plan and some recipes for you to try. It also includes nutritional and herbal therapy to help treat various medical problems that you encounter in recovery.

The Truth About Addiction and Recovery: The Life-Process Program for Outgrowing Destructive Habits, by Stanton Peele, Ph.D., and Archie Brodsky, with Mary Arnold. New York: Simon & Schuster, 1991.

With the Life-Process Program, you assess the impact that addiction has on your life. Then you take a look at what's really important to you. By doing this, you can answer the question, "Do I need to make a change?" If the answer is yes, the book gives you a complete set of guidelines to help you change behavior, including "Life Skills" training. This book offers a lifestyle-change approach to quitting addictions, a type of approach that has proven extremely effective in many studies.

COUNSELING/PSYCHOTHERAPY

When you're feeling down or upset, what can be more helpful than a sympathetic ear? A good listener can comfort you, make you feel strong, and give you a sense that someone is on your side. What's more, a good therapy session can help you find solutions to your problems.

Counseling can help you with many kinds of problems. A certified addictions counselor can help you specifically with quitting drugs. Most counselors or psychotherapists can generally help you improve your emotional condition or specifically help you reduce anxiety, relieve depression, enrich your relationships with others, and improve your attitude toward yourself.

Today, most health insurance policies cover counseling and psychotherapy. As a result, more and more people have been trying it and getting good results. If you give it a try, you may find that it can be beneficial for you as well.

How do you find the right counselor? Be prepared to shop around. You want a counselor whom you feel compatible with, one you can talk to comfortably. Keep looking until you find one who definitely helps you.

GROUP THERAPY

How would you feel if you could share your feelings in a group and be accepted for what you are? Pretty good, right? That's because a group has a certain self-affirming influence on everyone in it.

Like psychotherapy, group therapy can help you with specific behaviors. For example, you can find groups to help you with stress reduction, groups for people who have lost a loved one, and groups for people with a serious disease such as cancer.

If the 12-step approach works for you, you can find an "anonymous" group for almost anything: Narcotics Anonymous, Alcoholics Anonymous, Codependents Anonymous, Gamblers Anonymous, Overeaters Anonymous, Sex Addicts Anonymous, Child Abusers Anonymous, and more. Also, in this chapter you learned about some alternative groups: Women for Sobriety, Men for Sobriety, Rational Recovery, SMART Recovery, Discovery Empowerment Groups, and Secular Organizations for Sobriety. Now here's another group that you could try: Re-evaluation Counseling (RC). RC groups teach peer counseling methods to its members so that each member acts as a co-counselor. (For information, contact The International Re-evaluation Counseling Communities, "Recovery and Re-emergence," 719 2nd Ave. N., Seattle, WA 98109; phone 206-284-0311.) Otherwise, to access different types of psychotherapy groups, check with local mental health clinics and psychotherapists in private practice.

If given a chance, the right group can open you to parts of yourself that you haven't seen before. The right group can help you feel safe about yourself around others. Also, the right group can help you solve problems about yourself that will improve your overall approach to life. When you think about it, it might be worth your time to find some kind of group therapy that's just right for you.

When seeking a group, follow the same rules as for finding a counselor or therapist. Shop around for a group that focuses specifically on your problems, one in which you feel comfortable, and one that will help you grow.

LIGHT THERAPY

The sun's energy is what makes life on earth possible. Light from the sun spurs important biochemical processes, for example photosynthesis in plants and the production of vitamin D in humans.

Sunlight has been linked to human emotions. One example is happiness. A normal amount of natural sunlight, on a regular basis, promotes happiness. The less sunlight people get, the more depressed they become. Without natural full-spectrum lighting, work performance decreases, erratic behavior and nervousness increase, and the likelihood of disease is greater (everything from routine headaches to life-threatening cancers).

What kind of light causes problems? Any kind that deviates too much from the natural full-spectrum light given off by the sun. For instance, almost any kind of indoor (artificial) lighting causes problems. This includes conventional electric lightbulbs and almost all fluorescent lighting.

More than a hundred studies have shown that people do better at almost any task—and report feeling better—under full-spectrum lighting as opposed to any other form of lighting. Most artificial lighting concentrates in only one or two bands of the spectrum. Full-spectrum lighting blends all bands of the spectrum.

Of course, sunlight is the best (and original) source of full-spectrum lighting. Plan to expose yourself to some sunlight every day—not too much, maybe about a half-hour a day. You don't even have to sit directly in the sun—indirect sunlight works fine. This means that you can sit in the shade of a porch or under a tree and still gain the benefits. Get outside even when it's cold. You might be bundled up but the sun still dances in your eyes. A daily dose of sunlight does wonders for your disposition. Try it; you'll see.

Aside from enjoying natural sunlight, make sure to change your indoor lighting. For full-spectrum lighting, try Verilux, Inc. (for a catalog, write to P.O. Box 2455, Stamford, CT 06906, or call 888-544-4865). Or you can buy Chromolux full-spectrum light bulbs, manufactured by Lumiram Electric Corporation, in stores that carry health products.

EXPRESSIVE ARTS THERAPY

Drug addiction stifles creativity. Studies show that creativity—the ability for creative thought—diminishes in moderate to heavy drug users. However, when you quit using, your creativity will gradually return. So, as you recover, you need to channel your newfound creativity. It's there, waiting to be tapped. You can use it to help you make money or simply to enjoy yourself.

Some addiction recovery centers have now added artistic expression as a vital part of treatment. The reason: It has become a proven component of successful recovery. You can participate in a program at one of these centers, take various classes in your local community, or work with your creativity on your own.

First decide how you want to channel your creative energy. What form of artistic expression do you like? Drawing, painting, sculpting, pottery, crafts, photography, music, writing (including journal writing), dance, acting? Each one gives you an outlet and will help you feel more fulfilled. Each one offers the opportunity to express something deep inside you.

Choose one or more. Then get into it. Let your creativity flow. Don't hold back. Show your emotions through your form of artistry. Enjoy the freedom of creative expression.

HUG A FRIEND

Your sense of touch has a profound effect on your emotional life. Ever notice how a friendly touch can warm you? Touch someone and see. The feel of another person can be calming and reassuring. A simple hug reduces stress.

After working with drug addicts and alcoholics for over 50 years, Dr. Eugene Scheimann decided that people become addicted to drugs or alcohol as a substitute for touch. Addiction happens when we feel "out of touch," when we feel that we can't give or get the physical affection we need.

What can we do? Try any of the following:

Trading massages with a friend or loved one

Holding hands with your lover in the movies or on a walk

Hugging a friend

Patting your buddy on the back

Kissing and hugging your loved ones—whenever and as often as you can

This is therapeutic touch at its best. It's intimate. It's personal. It has the power of love and friendship behind it. Of course, you can go for a professional massage or some other kind of hands-on therapy, and it will help, too.

But take your sense of touch out of the closet. Act as if every day is National Feel a Friend Day. Occasionally, for a change, pretend it's National Hug an Enemy

Whether You Like It or Not Day. Touch as many lives as you can.

RELIGION

More than 100 different religions exist in the world today. Each has its own beauty. Each one supports a certain lifestyle and offers its own unique wisdom to humankind.

Any of these religions could be right for you. Which one do you like? For starters, here's a list of major religions:

Buddhism

Christianity

Hinduism

Islam

Jainism

Judaism

Shintoism

Sikhism

Sufism

Taoism

Zen Buddhism

Zoroastrianism

You can also add many major religions of the ancient world, such as the early pantheistic religions of Greece, Rome, Egypt, and Mesopotamia, and there are dozens upon dozens of unique, deeply rich, tribal religions found all over North and South America, Asia, Australia, Africa, and on every major island.

You may want to check out some of these other religions, especially if you question your present religion. You may find one that better suits your temperament and lifestyle. But even if you don't, the search in itself can be rewarding.

Of course, you may want to return to your original faith, the religion of your youth. Many people who break their drug addictions become totally reabsorbed in their original faith. The reason: They find a sense of personal renewal. When asked what's different the second time around, many report that they finally found themselves "letting go." What do they mean by this? Letting go of their problems, letting go of their struggle, and giving in to faith. In NA, there's an expression that seems apt here: "Let go and let God."

So how do you feel about religion? Is it an experience you'll want to nurture?

The right religion can help you find peace and love, joy, and inner strength. Indeed, the experience can be truly beautiful. But there's one more thing: You'll discover that religion, by launching you into the spiritual realm, will help to set you free.

SPIRITUAL HEALING

You don't necessarily need religion to help you feel free. Many techniques that are designed to improve your spiritual growth can do it, too.

Drugs stifle spiritual growth. Most heavy users remain spiritually lost their entire drug-taking careers. It doesn't matter how old you are—when you start using drugs heavily, you stop growing spiritually. When you quit the drugs, spiritual growth begins again.

So be prepared for the change. Plan to pursue some form of spiritual growth soon after you quit using. Be prepared ahead of time to make some new spiritual connection.

Then, as you make the change, watch what happens. You begin to view the world through different eyes. A fundamental shift in attitude occurs. Deep inside, you experience a new verve for life. You gain a fresh view of the world and develop a revitalized commitment to life.

How will you make this change? You can get involved in religion or try a 12-step program, or use any of the following spiritual techniques:

Meditation and Meditative Techniques

Meditation: Meditation is usually performed in a seated, cross-legged posture. You clear the mind by focusing on one thing, such as your breath, a sound (mantra), an image (yantra), or nothingness.

Zazen/Zen meditation: This kind of meditation is often done in a kneeling position. You might focus on a koan (an illogical thought intended to break through the logical mind, such as "What is the sound of one hand clapping?"), or you might focus on dropping the mind, by letting go of each thought as it arises.

Zen archery: You don't shoot the arrow—the arrow shoots itself. You are merely a medium through which the shooting occurs.

Sufi whirling: This is a method of dancing by spinning like a top. Induces a deep meditative state.

Yoga sutras: The sutras include over a hundred separate techniques or little meditative tricks that help you gain a glimpse of ultimate reality. See any of the five volumes of *The Book of Secrets,* by Bhagwan Shree Rajneesh, or *The Yoga Sutras of Patanjali,* by M.N. Dvivedi.

Rajneesh meditations. Incorporating the best from East and West, Rajneesh developed about 20 powerful meditations designed to awaken your spiritual self. Each of these meditations takes about an hour to do, usually in three to five parts, alternating Western "active" exercise with Eastern "passive" meditation postures. The result: Exceptional relaxation, euphoria, peace, contentment, and feelings of at-one-ment. See *The Orange Book,* by Bhagwan Shree Rajneesh.

Prayer: This is often done in a kneeling position. Prayers help you connect with a higher power by directing your thoughts to that power. You might offer thanks, supplication, or devotion. You might request forgiveness or ask for help. Most moments of prayer are solemn and accompanied by a meditative state of mind.

Many Paths of Yoga

You may choose many techniques but have only one path. The path that you choose relates to your general outlook, or to a consistent pattern of behavior that works well for you. Over time, as you change, your path might change. Some examples of paths follow:

Hatha yoga: You work with, and gain mastery over, your breath, health, and physical body.

Bhakti: You gain mastery over love and devotion, opening you to a higher consciousness (a path for those who live more in the heart).

Jnana yoga: You use your power of intellect to learn possibilities, to sort through alternatives, and to gain knowledge. Sometimes it takes a great deal of knowledge to realize how useless knowledge really is (a path for those who live more in the mind).

Karma yoga: You become one with your work or principal activity. You reach contentment through creating and producing various positive changes in the world.

Tantra: This is a method of feeling at one with whatever you happen to be doing in any given moment. You totally immerse yourself in the details of each and every moment. You achieve ecstasy by living each moment now.

Rebirthing

By using visualization and special breathing techniques, you relive the moment of your birth. This time around, however, you undo all the fear and trauma that accompanied your original birth. After a successful rebirthing, you feel as if you've been born again, only with a greater love and acceptance than before. Check local holistic health centers or new age directories for certified rebirthing practitioners in your area.

The Art of Surrender

When you give yourself up, you can live anew. Think of your self for a moment—think of everything you imagine your self to be. Now give it up. Throw this self away. It means nothing. Without this self demanding things, you have nothing to fight for, nothing to fear. As a result, you accept life and feel at one with it.

So, a new different self, a more accepting self, begins to emerge. But keep in mind that if this self becomes selfish and demanding, if it wants to take over your life and the lives of others, drop it. Even though this new self might be fighting for a "good cause," a better cause than your former self, drop it. Surrender it, too. Every time a self becomes fixated on something and begins to claim too much, move on. Leave it. That way, you'll continue to grow.

CHARITY/ALTRUISM

Do a good deed. When you help someone out, really help someone, you begin to feel warm inside. Your heart glows while you settle into a moment or two of peaceful contentment.

Try it. You don't just create these feelings in your mind. They're real. An actual change takes place inside. You not only feel better emotionally but become stronger physically. In a study of 2,700 people over a 10-year period, researchers found that doing regular volunteer work, more than any other activity, increased life expectancy.

In addition, offering a helping hand might actually help to heal you. In his bestselling book *Love, Medicine and Miracles,* Dr. Bernie Siegel reports that doing something for someone else boosts immune system activity. Indeed, compared to all options, it's among the best immune system boosters available.

It all comes down to one simple act: giving. So give some of your time, give some of your energy, and give some of the fruits of your labor to help another. It's bound to make you smile.

The Boy Scouts have a good slogan: "Do a good turn daily." You might want to make it your slogan, too. Meanwhile, keep in mind another popular slogan: "Helping You Helps Me."

GROWING IN LOVE

Love is the ultimate opening of the heart. Love means relationships, caring, giving, bhakti yoga, family, and togetherness.

God is love. Love brings spiritual awakening, and any spiritual awakening brings love.

When you open in love, you begin to bloom. You offer your "self" completely, without reservation. In truth, the self dissolves—it melts into the object of your affection. This is a love of total giving. This is a love that frees you from your psychic chains.

A selfish love won't do. A possessive love won't do. These are neurotic forms of love—destructive, draining, and incomplete.

The love of giving, the love that's pure of heart, can be for another person. It can be for God. It can be your love for all other people, for all living things, or for the entire universe.

It is an opening of the heart, a giving of the self, a maturing. It releases the true self, an uncluttered self, a selfless self, the self of the soul. Some brilliance from deep within comes shining through.

Allow yourself love. Let go into it. Free yourself within it. Open yourself to all the world.

To get a better feel for love, read *Love,* by Leo Buscaglia; *Loving Relationships,* by Sondra Ray; and *Love Is Letting Go of Fear,* by Gerald Jamplonsky.

Meanwhile, here's a parting thought on the subject of love:

> *Love and the self are one and the discovery of either is the realization of both.*

> —from Love, *by*
> Leo Buscaglia

Worksheet #7

Which Techniques Will You Do?

Instructions. Study the following groups. Then choose at least one technique from each group.

Select only techniques that you will do. *Then do them.* Plan to be doing all six techniques by the end of your second month away from drugs. (Do more than six techniques, if you want, by choosing any additional techniques that you would like to do.)

Group 1

- ☐ Acupuncture/CES
- ☐ Massage
- ☐ Biofeedback
- ☐ Bodywork/body movement
- ☐ Hypnosis

Group 2

- ☐ Autogenic training/self-hypnosis
- ☐ Visualization
- ☐ Affirmations
- ☐ Subliminal suggestion

Group 3

- ☐ A clinic or a live-in program
- ☐ Solitude and self-reflection
- ☐ Healing with laughter
- ☐ Turn off the television

Group 4

- ☐ Fasting
- ☐ Intestinal cleansing
- ☐ Herbal remedies
- ☐ Aromatherapy
- ☐ Homeopathy
- ☐ Chiropractic
- ☐ A chemical deterrent to drug use
- ☐ Alternative approaches to quitting drugs
- ☐ Counseling/psychotherapy
- ☐ Group therapy

Group 5

- ☐ Light therapy
- ☐ Expressive art therapy
- ☐ Hug a friend

Group 6

- ☐ Religion
- ☐ Spiritual healing
- ☐ Charity/altruism
- ☐ Growing in love

PART THREE

QUITTING AND MAKING IT WORK FOR YOU

CHAPTER 10

Okay, Pick a Day

Nothing is so perfectly amusing as a total change of ideas.

—Lawrence Sterne

Now it's time to take action. It's time to quit the drugs and begin to use everything you've learned so far.

Ever been in jail? The drug addiction is like being in jail. You're stuck—locked in. You've lost your freedom. But there's an interesting twist. You have the key! You have the key to your own jail cell. All you have to do is let yourself out. By quitting the drugs, you let yourself out.

By now you're probably looking forward to it. Physically, you need the change. Emotionally, you're ready.

Plus you've got all the information you need to be successful. If you quit using now and do all the things you've learned so far, you won't even think about the drugs. If you can do just half the things you've learned, that's still enough to guarantee your success.

Here's what you'll do in this chapter:

1. Review your Master Plan—all the things you'll do to help you when you quit.

2. Make a promise to quit using drugs.

3. Sign a contract to quit.

4. Pick a day and quit the drugs on that day.

By the end of this chapter, you'll free yourself from drugs and start a brand-new life.

USE EVERYTHING YOU'VE LEARNED SO FAR

A little knowledge might be a dangerous thing, but the right amount can help you move mountains. Right now you have enough knowledge to quit using drugs and to begin moving mountains. By way of a simple review, Worksheet #8 shows the most important changes you need to make. Use it to jog your memory.

Worksheet #8

Your Master Plan

Instructions. Review the key elements in your program for quitting. Check each one you have begun. Begin doing anything you haven't yet started.

☐ Stop denying the problems caused by drugs (Chapter 3, Worksheet #1).

☐ Look at the problems again. Remember how much you would like to avoid these problems (Chapter 4, Worksheet #3).

☐ Remember your reasons for quitting. Carry with you a written list of your most important reasons (Chapter 4, Worksheet #4).

☐ Follow your decision about NA (Chapter 5, Worksheet #5).

☐ Remember your alternatives to using drugs. Start doing them the day you quit (Chapter 6, Checklist #2).

- ☐ Change your diet (Chapter 7, Practice #4).
- ☐ Start your exercise program (Chapter 8, Practice #5).
- ☐ Use your relaxation techniques (Chapter 8, Checklist #3).
- ☐ Become more assertive (Chapter 8, Practice #6).
- ☐ Reduce stress (Chapter 8, Checklist #4).
- ☐ Talk with a friend (Chapter 8, Practice #7).
- ☐ Start additional techniques to renew yourself (Chapter 9, Worksheet #7).

PROMISE SOMEONE

The next important step is to promise someone close to you that you'll quit the drugs. Do it in writing.

Choose someone who is very close to you—a family member, a lover, or a friend—preferably someone who has urged you to quit using, someone who wants you to get better. Write this person a letter promising that you'll quit using. (Note: if you can't think of anyone, do this exercise by making a promise to yourself.)

Tell that person your most important reason for quitting. Say that you'll quit using soon and promise that you'll stay away from the drugs after you quit. Explain that you want to begin enjoying your life and not continue to ruin it. Affirm that you want to gain all the benefits of a drug-free lifestyle.

Write down all of this and make a copy of it. Give the original to a friend, lover, or family member. Put the copy under your pillow.

MAKE A CONTRACT

Here's a quick and simple way to put more power into your commitment: Promise yourself that you'll do it.

Make a vow to yourself that you'll stick to it. Make it your solemn oath. Then write it in a contract.

This last idea is perhaps the most important. When you write your vow into a contract and sign it, it becomes formal. It becomes a solid plan. It gives you something to live up to.

Worksheet #9

Contract to Quit Using Drugs

Instructions. You may use the following contract as is, or you can rewrite it in your own words. If you want to rewrite it, do that now. When you pick your date to quit, put that in your contract and sign it. In addition, you may choose someone close to you to witness your contract. This can be very helpful, but make sure to choose someone who will offer you encouragement.

It's a good idea to make a copy of your contract and hang it on your wall where you'll see it every morning.

Contract

I, _____ (name) promise to stop using _____ (name of drug or drugs) on _____ (date). I promise to follow my Master Plan to ensure my success.

I will use the techniques that I've learned in *How to Quit Drugs for Good.* I'll review my progress regularly and strengthen my commitment each day.

I will treat this contract as a solemn oath, as my vow, my personal commitment to myself.

Date: _____ Signed: _____
Witness: _____
(Optional)

*Some optional lines you can add to your contract:
I will not use drugs just for today.
I will not use drugs for this very minute.
I promise that if my heart is beating, I will not use.

PICK A DAY AND QUIT

Now you can get down to business. It's time. If you quit the drugs today and use everything you've learned so far, you'll succeed.

Admittedly, it won't be easy at first. You'll have to make a lot of changes all at once. But you can do it. Remember: Millions of people have quit using drugs successfully—and most of them had less practical information than you have.

Say When

The day you quit can be of key importance. By choosing your own day, you stay in control. You can take a little time to plan for it. You can get in the right frame of mind.

People who don't plan tend to quit after a horrible experience, like after a bout with the drugs that shows beyond a doubt how serious their problems really are. Maybe they nearly got killed. Maybe they hurt someone badly or woke up in jail or had to be hospitalized with serious medical complications.

If any of these happen—just once—it's too much. Don't wait for it to happen to you. It's like flirting with death. It might kill you.

You don't have to wait for a drug-induced tragedy to jar you awake. You already know all the problems caused by using drugs, and you know how serious these problems are. Why wait for them to get worse? Look at it this way: If you knew you had cancer and you knew the cure, would you wait for the cancer to spread more before starting the cure?

So, when should you quit? As soon as possible. You're ready. You're as ready as you'll ever be. Your body needs a break, and there's no better time than now to get your life in order.

If you need inpatient care for detox, plan for it. Tell people and arrange for your responsibilities to be taken care of. Take vacation or sick leave from work and enter a detox center.

Even if you don't go for inpatient care, take a couple of weeks off. You'll find that things go easier if you drop your normal routine.

In addition, please keep this in mind: Quitting is serious business. If you approach it seriously, you'll be stronger and more committed to getting good results. For this reason, don't bet money—it can put undue pressure on you—and don't make any grand announcements. Don't go around telling *everyone* that you're going to quit. This adds pressure, too. When it's your time to quit, do so quietly.

Now ask yourself this question: "What's the best time—in the near future—for me to quit the drugs?" Pick one day out of the next 30 days. Next week? Two weeks from now? The last weekend of the month? Make your date and stick to it.

Worksheet #10

Your Day

Instructions. Write the day and date you choose to quit using drugs. You may use drugs the day before you quit, but on the date you choose, you will not use. Then, every day thereafter, you will not use.

What day of the week did you pick? _____

What is the date (month/day/year)? _____

Now put the date that you'll quit using drugs in your contract—and sign it.

CHAPTER 11

Getting a Successful Start

Toto, I have a feeling we're not in Kansas anymore.

> —*Dorothy, in* The Wizard of Oz

Are you ready to soar into the stratosphere? If you were a rocket ship ready to be launched, a group of experts would clear you. "All systems go," they would say—each in their turn—when asked if you were ready for take-off.

You can use this technique on yourself. When you quit using drugs, immediately you need to clear yourself on three points:

1. How to cope with urges.
2. How to keep the right distance between you and drugs.
3. What to say when offered drugs.

In the three sections of this chapter, you'll check yourself on these important points.

COPING WITH URGES

It's going to happen. Every so often you'll get the urge to use. What will you do about it? How many ways do you know to help you cope with this urge?

How about 172? That's right. You know 172 ways to reduce, eliminate, or change the urge to use. In Checklist #2 (Chapter 6), you learned 120 alternatives to using drugs. In Checklist #4 (Chapter 8), you learned 22 surefire stress reducers. In Chapter 9, you studied 30 healing techniques.

Pick one. Do any of the healing techniques, any of the stress reducers, or any of your alternatives to using drugs, and you'll forget your desire to use. Or try any of the following five ways to cope with urges:

1. Outlast it: An urge remains strong for only five to 10 minutes. Simply wait it out.

2. View it as a power play that you can win: Don't let an urge take control. Fight it. Show that you're more powerful. Get mad at the urge if you need to. Argue with it. Get in control. Win.

3. Cut out sweets and caffeine: If you keep consuming sugar foods, you'll keep craving drugs, especially downers. Also, if you keep overdoing it with caffeinated beverages, you'll continue to crave drugs, especially uppers. Break your habits to sugar and caffeine—you'll feel much better.

4. Change your routine: People often use drugs as part of a routine, such as getting up in the morning, gathering together with a certain group of friends, or listening to a certain piece of music. So break any routine that you associate with using. Instead of following your same morning ritual, do something completely dif-

ferent. Instead of hanging with the same old friends in the same old places, find new friends in new places. Instead of listening to music that brings back memories of using drugs, listen to something new.

5. Use mind over matter: You can actually talk yourself out of an urge by looking at the facts. Remember how bad your life had gotten before quitting the drugs. Compare that to the life you have now—and consider the benefits you've gained by not using. Remember your worst high—think of the trouble you caused yourself or someone else. Think about how bad it really was. Then consider this: No matter how bad things get now, you can always make them worse by using. This viewpoint can help you make a powerful decision to stay away from the drugs.

Worksheet #11

---

177 Ways to Cope with Urges

Instructions. Review your favorite methods of coping (see Checklist #2, Chapter 6; Checklist #4, Chapter 8; Worksheet #7, Chapter 9; and the five ways listed above). Now pick your favorite 20 ways to cope with urges. Write each of these in your notebook or on a separate piece of paper. Review them often and use them whenever necessary.

HOW CLOSE CAN YOU GET TO DRUGS?

When you quit using, immediately your relationship with drugs changes. For a moment, think of your favorite drug as a person. You were in love with this person. In fact, you had an intimate relationship. But this person treated you badly. Very badly. This person hurt you emotionally and abused you physically.

Now you've broken the relationship. You've escaped. You're free. So what happens next?

Perhaps your emotion turns from love to hate. Maybe you hate this drug now. Maybe you prefer to avoid having this drug anywhere near you.

Or maybe you can part as "friends." Maybe you and your drug can't get along in a close relationship—you know you can't touch each other—but maybe you can be in the same room together.

It's up to you to decide.

Now that you've quit using this drug, what's your new relationship with it? How close can you get to it without being tempted to use?

Practice #8

Avoiding Temptation

Instructions. Consider each question carefully, then answer it. If you have any doubts, leave it blank. If you know you can handle a situation, check the box in front of the question. (If you're breaking addictions to more than one drug, do this complete practice for each drug.)

☐ Can you hold some of this drug in your hand without being tempted?

☐ Can you smell this drug (or the smoke from it) without being tempted?

☐ Can a family member or friend use this drug near you without tempting you?

☐ Can you go to a party and watch people using this drug without being tempted?

- ☐ Can you touch the paraphernalia (pipes, syringes, roach clip, and so on) without being tempted?
- ☐ Can you see the paraphernalia without being tempted?
- ☐ Can you watch people using this drug on a movie or television show without being tempted?
- ☐ Can you tell doctors that you've been addicted to this drug and ask them not to prescribe any medication that would jeopardize your recovery?
- ☐ Can you walk or drive past the places where you got high without wanting to go in?
- ☐ Can you walk or drive past the places where you used to buy this drug without wanting to buy?

How close can you get?

If you think you'll have trouble with a situation, avoid it. Avoid it any way you can.

Make plans to avoid it. Make excuses to avoid it. If you can't avoid a certain situation, leave early. Get away from this situation as soon as you feel the least bit uncomfortable. Meanwhile, practice your reasons for not using drugs (Checklist #5, later in this chapter) and be ready to tell them to anyone at any time.

In addition, you can make a contract with yourself whenever you feel the need:

Contract Not to Use Drugs for a Specific Situation

I promise not to use _____ (name of drug or drugs) during _____ (specific situation) on _____ (date). I will remain levelheaded in the situation. And no matter what happens, I will choose not to use.
Signed: _____
Date: _____

And Remember: You Get Stronger and Stronger

When you first quit using drugs, many situations will seem hard for you. You'll often feel tempted to use. However. as time goes by, you'll feel tempted less and less. It doesn't take very long—especially when you work to improve your health. In a year or so, you'll find that you can experience most situations in Practice #8 without being tempted at all.

Just give yourself the time and allow things to change.

FOR ANYONE WHO ASKS YOU . . .

What will you say when someone asks, "Do you want to get high?" You can bet your life that many people will ask you. Do you know what to tell them?

When you quit using, it helps to have a few ways to say, "No thanks." It helps to have a few solid excuses for not using. You almost need to talk about each addictive drug in a whole new light. Instead of talking about how much you want it or need it, you need to talk about why you don't want it, why you don't need it, or why you can't have it.

Think about it. Do you know, for example, what you'll tell your friends? What will you say to a friend who urges you to get high? What will you tell your date tonight? What about your family—what will you tell them?

Try this: Say to yourself a few times, "I don't use drugs." Practice it. Say it silently. Now say it out loud a few times. To be more specific, state the name of the drug or drugs that you don't use. For example, "I don't do coke." "I don't smoke dope." "I don't shoot smack." "I don't pop pills."

Then, after you quit, repeat this phrase to yourself often, and be ready to repeat it to others whenever the issue arises. Also, you might try some of these variations:

No thanks, I don't use.

No, I quit using the stuff.

Thanks, but I don't do it anymore.

Oh, didn't you know—I don't do drugs.

When people ask, sometimes you'll give a reason for not using, sometimes you'll give an excuse.

A reason for not using tells why you don't use at all. A reason might tell people why you've quit and why you don't plan to use again. For example, "No thanks, I stopped the drugs because they were causing too many health problems."

An excuse covers you for one night or just for the moment. For example, "No thanks, I'd rather mingle with the guests." If you don't want to get into any personal details with people, you can simply make excuses. You can make excuses from now until your dying day—and never take another hit.

By the way, with excuses you can make up anything. An excuse doesn't have to be true—just effective. Have fun with it. Surprise people. Be outlandish. Laugh about it.

Checklist #5

Why I'm Not Using

Instructions. Review these *reasons* and *excuses* for not using drugs. Select any that you would feel comfortable using and put a check next to them.

Now go back through the list and put a second check next to those that you like the most. Write them on a separate piece of paper. These are your favorite reasons and excuses for not using. Practice them. Be ready to spring them on anyone, at any time, in any situation.

Reasons

☐ Drugs nearly killed me.

☐ _____ (name of drug) nearly killed me.

☐ I had to quit to save my life.

☐ My liver got so bad I had to quit.

☐ I have already gotten high enough in my life.

☐ I have already used as many drugs in my life as 10 normal people.

☐ I have already used enough drugs in my life to kill a normal person.

☐ I nearly got fired from work. I had to quit the drugs to save my job.

☐ I got very sick from _____ (name of drug), and I need to stay away from it so that I can heal myself.

☐ I had a bad scrape with the law and had to quit using to stay out of jail.

☐ The drugs were screwing me up totally—making me crazy. I had to quit.

☐ I was losing my mind with _____ (name of drug).

☐ I was having too many fights with my family (my parents, wife, husband, kids).

☐ I had to quit because I was afraid I might hurt someone.

☐ Things were really getting bad. I had to quit to turn my life around.

☐ The drugs were robbing me of energy. I could hardly do anything.

☐ _____ (name of drug) was making me a nervous wreck. I had to quit.

☐ I quit the drugs because I want to set a good example for my children. I really care about them.

☐ I quit using so that I could regain my health.

- ☐ The drugs were blocking my thinking. I quit so that I could think clearly again.
- ☐ I quit to gain control of my life.
- ☐ I needed to get free. I felt like the drugs were holding me in a cage.
- ☐ I needed to regain my creativity.
- ☐ I needed to avoid pancreatitis.
- ☐ I had to reduce my blood pressure.
- ☐ I was using so much it caused internal bleeding.
- ☐ I had to quit.
- ☐ I had severe hypoglycemia and had to quit.
- ☐ I had _____ (serious physical condition) and had to quit to save myself.
- ☐ _____
- ☐ _____
- ☐ _____
- ☐ _____

Excuses

- ☐ No, thanks, I'm the designated driver tonight.
- ☐ No, thanks, I just had one. (Feel free to lie. Any excuse is okay, as long as it keeps you from using.)
- ☐ No thanks, I'm fine.
- ☐ No thanks, I'm high as a kite already. (Remember that you can make up any lie you want.)
- ☐ No thanks, I'm out of my mind as it is.
- ☐ Things are bad enough. I would only make them worse by using.
- ☐ My doctor said I had to quit the stuff.
- ☐ I can't touch a spot of it. I'm taking naltrexone.
- ☐ I would rather mingle with the guests.
- ☐ I would rather dance.
- ☐ I can't do any tonight. I have too much to do tomorrow.
- ☐ No, thanks, I have to get up early tomorrow.

☐ No, thanks, I was just leaving.

☐ No, thanks, I'm not using today.

☐ Not today. I need a day off from the stuff.

☐ No thanks, I promised _____ that I wouldn't use today.

☐ I promised myself that I wouldn't use today, and I'm going to keep my promise.

☐ It's done me in. I couldn't handle another hit (or snort, sip, shot, pill).

☐ My _____ (sickness or internal problem) has been acting up and I can't touch the stuff today.

☐ No, thanks, I'm just doing this fruit juice instead. It's getting me high.

☐ No, I'm not using, just for today.

☐ Can't you tell? I've become a teetotaler—give me a cup of tea.

☐ Just for the hell of it, I'm not using today.

☐ Maybe you expected me to say yes, but no, I don't want any today. Thanks anyway.

☐ Not right now, thanks.

☐ I can't possibly do any right now. And I can't even begin to tell you why. Just go ahead and I'll catch you later.

☐ It seems to bother you that I'm not using. You keep asking me to do some. If it bothers you that much, I'd better be going. See ya.

☐ No thanks, I don't use.

☐ _____

☐ _____

☐ _____

☐ _____

CHAPTER 12

15 Common Problems and How to Solve Them

All things are difficult before they are easy.
—*Thomas Fuller, M.D.*

When breaking an addiction to drugs, 15 common problems arise. Everyone experiences them, but by knowing what to expect, you can be prepared.

Two kinds of problems occur: (1) those that drugs caused and (2) those that drugs concealed. The problems that drugs caused relate to physical health. As a general rule, the more drugs you used, the more you compromised your health. For these kinds of problems, you need to revitalize your body and give it time to heal.

The problems that drugs concealed relate to emotions. These are the emotional problems that you never really faced, the real life problems that drugs helped you forget. When you quit the drugs, they reappear.

Now it's time to face both kinds of problems. It's time to stop hiding, time for you to confront your problems head-on—and resolve them without drugs.

The following descriptions tell you what to expect and give you some realistic ways to resolve each problem.

ANXIETY

Feel nervous? Tense? That's a normal reaction to quitting drugs. The drugs had your nervous system overstimulated or oversedated for a long time. When you take the drugs away, your nervous system gets highly active.

What's worse, if you used the drugs to calm yourself whenever you felt tense, now instead the tension comes through full force. How will you cope with it now that you can't use the drug?

First, remember diet. Cut out all sweets. Don't even use artificial or substitute sweeteners. And cut out caffeine. Second, get a lot of exercise. Exercise relieves tension. Third, use stress reduction techniques. Especially try yoga or other forms of bodywork and body movement. Other possibilities are acupuncture, massage, biofeedback, herbal remedies, and aromatherapy. All can help reduce anxiety.

DEPRESSION

Everyone experiences some sadness in life and seeks ways to cope with it. Heavy drug users use the drugs to cope. Maybe you used drugs to forget some of your sad memories.

Also, most drugs stimulate the pleasure centers in the brain by increasing the efficiency of the biochemical dopamine. However, when you quit using the drugs, your brain will show dopamine deficits for a long time.

When you stop using, you must face your sadness head-on. Now is your time to deal with it in a realistic manner.

What works? Exercise. A brisk walk or a highly active workout relieves depression. Yoga does the same and increases your mental power as well. What else? Talk with a friend or counselor. Use visualization, affirmations, or self-hypnosis. Turn off the television. Or try light therapy, expressive art therapy, and charity (doing something for others). In your diet, stay away from sweets.

ANGER

The moderate to heavy use of drugs causes anger. Now that you've quit the drugs, you probably get less angry, although you might still have some problems with this intense emotion. Most likely, you'll find that anger has its emotional roots deep in your childhood. For this reason, counseling, psychotherapy, or group therapy might help.

Otherwise, you can alter the biochemical triggers to your anger. For example, overeating and too much caffeine are the two most common triggers. If you eat too much—especially if you eat too much animal food—or drink too much coffee, you're easily prone to angry moods. If you cut back your food consumption and eliminate meat and caffeine from your diet, you can virtually eliminate anger.

How else can you deal with anger? Any form of exercise, bodywork, or body movement technique will help, as will visualization techniques. Solitude can help (alone, you can even yell out loud as a way to get your anger out). Or you can channel your rage through expressive arts therapy. Or try fasting—even one day can change your entire perspective.

DISTURBED SLEEP

Drug use disrupts sleep. It blocks dreams and reduces restfulness. That's why, on the average, moderate to heavy users need more sleep than nonusers.

Even after you quit the drugs, it takes a long time before your sleep assumes a normal pattern. This will take at least a few months or even as long as a year.

How will you be affected? You might have insomnia, or you might have trouble getting up in the morning. Also, you'll probably dream excessively.

Further, many of your dreams will be extremely lucid. The most common theme for these lucid dreams? Drug use. For example, you'll dream that you've lost control and started using again. Or you'll dream that you've gotten high and maybe gotten in some kind of trouble. These dreams will bother you, and you'll wake with a start. The dream will seem so real that it will take you five or 10 minutes to realize that the events didn't happen.

What can you do about disrupted sleep? Exercise does wonders. Daily active exercise will make you naturally tired when it's time to sleep. Doing yoga stretches at night will help you relax into a deep sleep, and doing it in the morning will cure your grogginess. These are the two favored times to do yoga. Other hints: Stop watching television and start using relaxation techniques, such as autogenic training. Also, try herbal remedies or aromatherapy.

GUILT

Most moderate to heavy drug users experience guilt over things that they've done while high—and usually for good reason. Very often, they've done something embarrassing, something mean, or something harmful to themselves or others.

When you stop getting high, you don't do all those stupid or horrible things that made you feel guilty. So already you've made a big change.

Nevertheless, you'll still feel guilty over some things. Most of this guilt will be over normal everyday affairs. Yet even this will diminish as time goes on and you start doing more and more things to feel proud about.

One thing to remember: Drop the guilt that you feel for your past mistakes. Don't feel guilty for all the terrible things you did while high on drugs. Don't feel guilty for things you did in childhood before you ever started getting high. What helps? First, make amends to anyone you feel you've harmed. Work as hard as you can to correct any mistakes you've made. Each day, take some of your time to make it up to people, to make things right again. Once you're doing this, you can drop the guilt. Drop it. Drop it completely. You can't change it anyway. You can only change yourself in the present, and you're doing the best you can right now.

For extra help, try "people therapies": talk with a friend or counselor, get into group therapy (including any recovery group), or do some kind of volunteer or charity work. Also, use your assertiveness skills so that you won't feel guilty about the way you talk to people. Or dissolve your guilt with laughter. Or meditate. In meditation, you drop all thoughts of the past and of the future.

OVEREATING

When you quit any addiction, you tend to overeat. Your body replaces excesses of one thing by consuming excesses of another. When you quit the drugs, you'll probably feel hungry all the time and you might start overeating. This will continue for a few months at least, maybe as long as a year and a half, until your body balances itself.

One way to approach overeating: Simply allow it. Allow yourself to eat all the time, but eat only vegetables and fruit. Carry with you, at all times, carrot sticks, celery sticks, raisins, or apples. That way, when you do overeat, you won't gain weight; in fact, you'll probably lose weight.

Also, try fasting to adjust your internal balance. And do exercise of all kinds. Exercise burns the calories from food and helps your body digest food more efficiently.

GASTROINTESTINAL DISTRESS

When you quit the drugs, it's very likely that you'll experience frequent constipation or diarrhea. Or you might experience both, one alternating with the other.

Constipation is normal. It happens whenever you break an addiction to any kind of drug or food, such as alcohol, nicotine, caffeine, or sugar. It's part of your body's natural healing process. Constipation occurs as your intestinal muscles return to normal, operating on their own without the influence of whatever addictive substance you just quit.

All the drugs of abuse cause many health problems in the intestines. Many of these problems, such as colitis and Crohn's disease, lead to diarrhea. So after you quit the drugs, you'll probably have diarrhea until your body can heal itself.

How can you help the healing process? Diet is one of the best ways. Eat whole grains, beans, vegetables, and fruit, all of which are high in fiber. Avoid meat, milk and milk products, white-flour products, and fruit juices. Exercise helps, too. A long walk does wonders. Hatha yoga helps to heal all the organs, including the intestines. Also, you might try a colonic to clean your intestines (no more than one or two a year), or use herbal remedies or fasting to regularize your entire system.

VISIONS/HALLUCINATIONS

When you first quit the drugs, you might have serious hallucinations. You know about this if you've ever experienced severe withdrawal symptoms or delirium tremens (DTs). Hallucinations almost always accompany the convulsive shaking of DTs. For example, people might see snakes, worms, or insects crawling all over their bodies and think they're absolutely real.

These hallucinations can literally scare you to death. They can seem so real and frightening that you may do something fatal. However, after a few days the hallucinations disappear.

Whether or not you experienced hallucinations during the first few days of withdrawal, you might have mild hallucinations that can last for a few months afterward. What are mild hallucinations? They seem like visions. They come to you as lucid dreams, only they happen when you're awake. For example, you might have visions of dead relatives coming back to help you. You might see religious figures reaching out to help you. Or you might envision yourself struggling to get free from some archetypal villain (such as the devil) or someone from your long-ago past who was a bad influence on you.

What to do? Allow it—experience it. The visions and hallucinations dispel emotionally charged material stored deep within you. It's part of your long-term mental and emotional healing. So, as much as possible, take an active role in the process. You can use visualization techniques to guide your visions toward the positive. You can use affirmations to strengthen your mental imagery. You can use these to become your own guide in wonderland.

FUZZY THINKING

You might not have visions or hallucinations after you quit the drugs, but you're bound to have problems with fuzzy thinking. This can last for the first two months to as long as two years after you quit. What's fuzzy thinking? It's the inability of the mind to grasp a thought or idea, resulting in confused expression and communication. It can happen with all thoughts, or it can happen with specific types of thoughts.

Fuzzy thinking affects anyone who uses drugs. The reason? Drugs interrupt the brain's neurochemistry, interfering with thought formulation and thought transmission. When you stop using drugs, it takes a long time to restore the balance of your neurochemical functioning.

But you can do it. What's more, you can get your brain functioning better than it ever functioned in your entire life—even better than it functioned before you started with the drugs. (This applies, of course, only to the parts of your brain that still function. Any parts with physical or organic damage from drug abuse might remain dysfunctional.)

How can you cure fuzzy thinking? The "big two": diet and active exercise. In diet, stay away from sugars, caffeine, nicotine, alcohol, chemical additives (including artificial sugars), and any kind of drugs, including over-the-counter drugs. Other helpful hints: Turn off the television. Also, try yoga, acupuncture, massage, bodywork/body movement, fasting, intestinal cleansing, or chiropractic.

THE SAME OLD FAMILY SITUATION

Quitting drugs produces another problem. When you change, and your family doesn't, what happens? Tension. Your change will be hard on family members because it means that they have to change, too.

By quitting the drugs, you become responsible more often. You become more mature. You are less often a dependent child and less often a vicious monster. Yet people in your family have gotten used to helping the dependent child in you or running from the vicious monster. Now what do they do?

Many marriages end when a drug using partner doesn't change, but almost as many end after a drug using partner stops using. Why? Sometimes drug users change so much after quitting that they alienate their spouses. All of a sudden, the spouse is living with a stranger—a mature stranger, but a stranger nonetheless. And this reaction is often felt by the ex-user's children, parents, and extended family. The old, dependent, drugged-out "you" has died, and a new "you" has replaced it.

What can you do to ensure your acceptance and to help those around you? Practice assertive behavior. Tell family members exactly who you are now and exactly how you feel. Give them plenty of time to accept the new you. And you need to allow them plenty of time to change their ways, too. Also, try family counseling. It can be very effective at helping family members break out of old patterns of relating. 12-Step Groups can also help (NA for you; Families Anonymous, Co-Anon Family Groups, Nar-Anon Family Groups, and Codependents Anonymous for your spouse and children). Other alternatives you might try: sharing religion together, spiritual healing, or "growing in love" groups, including relationships training.

SEX

Moderate to excessive use of drugs causes sexual dysfunction in both men and women. And when you quit using, it doesn't get better immediately. It takes time. In fact, it often gets worse before it gets better. This problem can take a few months to a year to improve, depending on the seriousness of your dysfunction.

To speed the healing, try yoga. It's probably the single most effective way to revitalize your sexuality. Regular physical exercise helps, too. And remember to eat a good diet—one free of sugar, nicotine, caffeine, and alcohol, all of which cause sexual problems on their own. Also try spiritual healing, sex counseling, sexual relationships training (including "growing in love" groups), and visualization (visualize yourself a sexually healthy person).

FRIENDS

You can expect changes in your relationships with friends after you quit the drugs. As with family members, anticipate that your friends will be more—or less—accepting of the new you.

When in doubt concerning your friendships, remember this important advice: Keep any friend who wishes you well after you've quit the drugs and drop any friend who tries to sabotage you. The first kind of friend is a real friend. The second kind, who can't accept the nonaddicted you, was never a friend in the first place.

Try to do at least as much for your friends as they do for you. That way, you'll keep them. And remember to give them hugs on a regular basis.

SETBACKS

It's going to happen. Everything will be going great. You'll feel on top of the world. Then there will be some problem, an unavoidable tragedy or some serious disappointment. Your world will seem to crumble, and all you'll want to do is get high.

Getting high will appear as the only way you know to handle the situation. That's because it's what you have so often done. Remember, you've spent a lot of time learning how to deal with problems by using drugs.

Now it's time to handle these tough situations without using. You can learn to do it. If you do it once, you can do it again. Just practice. It gets easier over time.

Meanwhile, keep this in mind when you get hit with a setback and feel like getting high: *No matter how bad things get, you can always make them worse by using drugs.*

SLIPS

Even though you know all that you know about quitting and being successful with it, you might still slip.

You might succumb to the lure of drugs and begin to use. What happens then? What happens if you do slip and begin to use? What happens if you keep using until you're down-and-out wasted? What happens if you keep getting high for a whole week?

Catch it. Stop it. Drop the drug use and start all over again. Get right back on your own program of not using (your program for recovery). Go back to Chapter 9 and pick it up from there.

Moreover, be sure to drop any guilt about making the slip. All is not lost. Look at it this way: You gained an experience. You learned something about your approach that didn't work.

It's easy enough to pick up where you left off. It's your inalienable right to continue toward your goal of becoming drug free. And just remember: You will be a success.

CELEBRATIONS/PARTIES

Many people know only one way to celebrate: by getting high. Without the drugs, how do you celebrate? How can you enjoy yourself at a party without getting high?

Parties pose a problem because they go hand in hand with the use of drugs and alcohol. People expect you to get a buzz. Also, parties and celebrations are a normal part of life. They happen all the time.

So what should you do? Find other ways to enjoy yourself. At a party, take time to talk to others. Get excited simply by hearing what people have to say. Lose yourself in the music. To celebrate some special occasion, have sex instead of drugs, take a nature hike instead of getting high, or do a little dance (whether there's music playing or not). Take time to do any of your favorite alternatives to using (Checklist #2, Chapter 6). Do anything but use.

Remember: You achieve more success in your life by staying away from drugs. So don't get high to celebrate—you'll only ruin your success.

If you enter into the spirit of celebration—without using drugs—you'll soon find that you have more fun. Allow yourself to become totally absorbed in the festive atmosphere. Instead of losing yourself in drugs, find yourself in the celebration. Remain aware—and enjoy it to the fullest.

CHAPTER 13

Enjoying the Benefits of Not Using

Every living creature, even a puppy,
is at the center of the universe.
—Anatole France

Quitting drugs is one of the best things that can happen to you. You gain many rewards: your health, your vitality, and your freedom. Now you can begin enjoying yourself.

In this chapter, you'll look on the bright side of quitting. You'll figure how much time and money you save. You'll set up a plan to give yourself rewards. And you'll evaluate all the great benefits you gain as a result of getting off the drugs.

TWO BIG BENEFITS

Most people like to hear how to save time or how to save money. How about you? When you quit using drugs, you'll save both time and money. In fact, you'll save a considerable amount of each.

It can be well worth it, as you'll see.

Worksheet #12

How Much Time Do You Save?

Instructions. How much time do you waste because of drugs? Fill in the number of hours for various activities.

Number of Hours   *In an Average Week*

+ _____   Amount of time spent high.

+ _____   Time spent getting high. (Count the time you spend getting to "your own special place," time securing your place—locking all doors and windows, closing shades, and so on—and time spent preparing everything for use.)

+ _____   Time spent making trips to the seller's location to score your drugs for the coming week. (Include time spent finding the seller, waiting for the seller, and time spent finding another seller because this one ran out.)

+ _____   Time spent making extra trips to the seller's location to buy "a little bit extra" because you ran out.

+ _____   Time spent withdrawing from drugs. (Count withdrawal time that was serious enough to keep you from doing something useful. Include any time lost from work.)

+ _____   Time spent thinking about using. (Time spent planning your day around drugs, debating with yourself when to start using each day, planning how to pace yourself and how to hide your drug use from others, and so on.)

+ _____   Time lost in nervousness as you try to postpone your first dose of the day; or, time lost in physical distress as you rush to get your first dose.

+ _____	Time lost sleeping. (Drugs cause people to need more sleep and to spend more time sleeping. After eight hours a night, count every extra hour you need as time lost due to drugs.)
= _____	Total hours per week lost due to drug use (add all the above numbers).
× 52	
= _____	Numbers of hours spent in the average year on the above.
+ _____	Each year: Time spent in court hearings and in jail for drug-related charges or in court-ordered programs.
+ _____	Each year: Time spent in hospitals due to accidents. Count accidents you had when high on drugs and accidents you had when withdrawing from drugs.
+ _____	Each year: Time spent in hospitals for medical complications due to drug use. Count also the time spent in recovery at home.
+ _____	Each year: Time spent repairing or replacing things you've damaged while high.
= _____	*Total number of hours lost each year due to drug use (add the five numbers above).

*You'll gain this many hours for yourself each year by quitting the drugs.

Worksheet #13

How Much Money Do You Save?

Instructions. How much money do you spend on drugs? Fill in the dollar amount for each kind of expenditure.

Amount
Spent   *In an Average Week*

+ $ _____	Buying drugs. (Count all illicit drugs that you buy in an average week.)

+ $ _____   Amount spent on gasoline to make trips to the various sellers you buy from.

+ $ _____   Amount spent on over-the-counter medications to help you feel better when you're high on, or withdrawing from, the illicit drugs.

+ $ _____   Amount spent on taxis to take you home when you're too high to drive.

+ $ _____   Amount spent buying drugs for other people.

+ $ _____   Amount spent on paraphernalia (papers, foil, pipes, clips, needles, and so on).

= $ _____   Total dollars spent per week on the drug habit. (Add all the above numbers.)

× 52

= $ _____   Dollars spent in an average year on all the above.

+ $ _____   In a year: Dollar value of items lost while high on drugs (lighters, car keys, makeup kits, jewelry, watches, umbrellas, hats, and so on.)

+ $ _____   In a year: Amount of money lost while high.

+ $ _____   In a year: If you've lost your license because of drug use, amount spent on taxis and other forms of transportation to help you get around while you don't have your license.

+ $ _____   In a year: Amount spent on fines to pay for drug-related legal problems. (Include amount spent for lawyers to defend you.)

+ $ _____   In a year: Amount spent on drug-related medical problems. (Include drug-related injuries due to falling, getting into fights, and so on.)

+ $ _____   In a year: Amount spent on things you've broken or wrecked while high on drugs (cars, clothing you've ruined, household items you've broken or torn up, damage due to fires you might have started while high, and so on).

+ $ _____   In a year: Amount of income lost because you can't hold a job.

+ $ _____   In a year: Amount of money lost working for a lower wage than what you're capable of earning. (Figure how much money you lose during an average year. For example, you might be working at a job for $5.00 an hour, but if you stayed away from drugs you could hold a more responsible position paying $12.00 an hour, which means that you're losing $14,560 each year.)

= $ _____   *Total amount lost each year due to drug use (add the above nine numbers).

*You'll have this much extra money each year by quitting the drugs.

YOU DESERVE A REWARD

You've undergone a major change: You've quit using drugs. This takes a lot of strength and a lot of effort. Now, what's in it for you?

Of course, you'll gain some natural benefits from quitting, benefits that unfold gradually, such as regaining your health, feeling better, and thinking more clearly. But you deserve even more.

Studies show that rewards for success reinforce the success. This means that if you reward yourself for staying off the drugs, you'll want to keep up the good work. A reward gives you a reason to continue.

And what can be more fun. You can choose something that you really like to do—and do it. You can buy something special for yourself, something you always wanted. You can treat yourself to little things more often.

Don't worry about spending extra time. Don't worry about spending extra money. You have plenty of each, now that you've quit the drugs. So go for it. Feel free.

Checklist #6

Claim Your Prizes

Instructions. Go through the list and choose any rewards that you would like to give yourself. Write any additional ideas in the blank lines. Then plan to give yourself these rewards on a regular basis for your continued success at not using drugs. Give yourself at least two rewards per week—*every week.* And enjoy them.

☐   Buy yourself a book.

☐   Subscribe to a magazine you like.

☐   Buy some new running shoes, hiking shoes, work boots, or new dress shoes.

☐   Buy yourself some new clothing (a dress, a shirt, a pair of slacks, a new hat).

☐   Buy some new fishing equipment.

☐   Buy a new tape or compact disc.

☐   Buy yourself a new set of work tools, a power tool that you've always wanted, or a new workbench.

☐   Buy some new camera equipment.

☐   Buy yourself a special piece of equipment to help with any hobby:

     ☐   An easel for art

     ☐   A pottery wheel

     ☐   A typewriter or word processor

     ☐   _____

     ☐   _____

     ☐   _____

☐   Write a poem.

☐   Get together with a friend.

☐   Go to a movie.

☐   Go out dancing.

☐   Go to a comedy club for an evening of laughter.

☐   Go out to dinner.

☐ Get a massage.

☐ Take a long walk.

☐ Take a special class.

☐ Get your hair styled.

☐ Listen to a piece of music.

☐ Read a book or magazine.

☐ Make a special meal.

☐ Call a friend for a long chat.

☐ Take a long bath with herbal bath oils.

☐ Take some time all to yourself to work on a craft or hobby you like.

☐ Take time to work on your favorite creative project (painting, sculpting, writing, music, photography).

☐ Work with any of the healing techniques you liked in Worksheet #7 (Chapter 9). You can go to a specialist, take classes, or study on your own. Write down what you'll do (for example, "Take a class to help me study spirituality").

    ☐ _____

    ☐ _____

    ☐ _____

☐ Other rewards you would like (for ideas, see Checklist #2, Chapter 6):

    ☐ _____

    ☐ _____

    ☐ _____

    ☐ _____

    ☐ _____

Treat yourself. You deserve it.

HAVING FUN

Have you noticed? Now that you've quit the drugs, things are changing. You're beginning to grow. You're beginning to feel better. Life suddenly seems worthwhile.

Have you seen the changes?

Generally, you become more responsible. You feel happier, healthier, and more optimistic. You begin to think more clearly, show more love, receive more love, know more, and become wiser and more mature. In short, your life is more successful.

How have you changed? Take a good look. Use the following worksheet as a guide.

Worksheet #14

The Benefits of Not Using

Instructions. Put a check next to the changes that you've made and the benefits that you've been enjoying by not using drugs. Consider how important these changes and benefits are to you. Remember them. Write them on a separate piece of paper and review them from time to time. Remind yourself over and over that the only way to get these benefits is to stay off the drugs.

☐ I'm getting healthy again.

☐ I have my health for the first time in my life.

☐ I don't have as many headaches.

☐ I don't have as many physical pains.

☐ My liver is healing (no pains in my right side anymore).

☐ My pancreas is healing (no pains in my left side anymore).

☐ My stomach isn't always hurting.

☐ My stomach isn't upset as often.

☐ My ulcer is going away.

☐ My digestion is improving.

- [ ] My bowel movements are becoming regular again.
- [ ] My blood pressure is becoming normal.
- [ ] My heart feels stronger (my chest pains are going away).
- [ ] My eyes are healing. I can see more clearly.
- [ ] I feel more limber.
- [ ] My muscles don't ache as much.
- [ ] I'm beginning to eat normally again.
- [ ] I'm beginning to lose weight and look more trim.
- [ ] My nerves are settling down. I'm not as nervous or tense anymore.
- [ ] I don't get angry as often.
- [ ] I don't get as angry as I used to.
- [ ] I don't feel violent anymore.
- [ ] I feel stronger inside.
- [ ] Sex is better.
- [ ] I can now have healthier babies.
- [ ] My concentration is better.
- [ ] My creativity is returning.
- [ ] I can think more clearly.
- [ ] My memory has returned.
- [ ] I feel good about myself.
- [ ] I'm getting more compliments from others.
- [ ] I look better physically.
- [ ] I'm getting to work on time.
- [ ] I feel confident that I can hold a job now.
- [ ] I feel comfortable driving. I don't have to worry about tickets, lawyers, fines, or losing my license.
- [ ] I can go out and have a good time without making a fool of myself.
- [ ] It feels good not having to sneak around, here and there, to use drugs.
- [ ] I feel more open than I used to.
- [ ] I feel like I can be more honest with people, including myself.

- [ ] I don't complain as much as I used to.
- [ ] I feel like I'm beginning to grow—like maybe my life can go somewhere now.
- [ ] I no longer feel like a loser.
- [ ] I have more money to spend on the things I want.
- [ ] I have a stronger sense of pride and accomplishment.
- [ ] I feel like I can make something out of myself, and I'm beginning to do so.
- [ ] I feel more organized now.
- [ ] I trust myself and my own judgment more.
- [ ] I don't feel as guilty about my behavior anymore.
- [ ] I'm more assertive now.
- [ ] I can communicate better.
- [ ] More and more, I can be around other people and feel comfortable with them.
- [ ] I'm less anxious.
- [ ] I feel more loving.
- [ ] I'm much better with my family.
- [ ] I'm resolving issues with my family.
- [ ] Now I go out more often with my family.
- [ ] I now have a more positive view about relationships with the opposite sex.
- [ ] My relationship with a sexual partner is getting better.
- [ ] My loving relationships are getting better.
- [ ] Relationships with my friends are getting better.
- [ ] More people seem to like me now.
- [ ] I feel that I can help others in certain ways, and I'm beginning to do so.
- [ ] In general, my life gets better and better.
- [ ] Lately, I'm enjoying myself more and more.

CHAPTER 14

Inspirations to Help Make Quitting Easy

The great art of life is how to turn the surplus life of the soul into life for the body.
                    —*Henry David Thoreau*

Here, you'll find music for the soul—harmonies of thoughts and feelings to help awaken your deep inner self. These are personal meditations—ideas that you can act on—to make your life go easier.

What's an inspiration?

Inspiration literally means "to breathe in." Each new breath bursts with oxygen, energy, and vitality. Breath continues life itself. Breath is soul-life—the life of the spirit.

Here are 10 inspirations. Each can be extremely helpful for anyone who has quit using drugs.

DO ONE THING AT A TIME

People who have quit using drugs often feel overwhelmed with too much to do. Their minds constantly juggle thoughts of five, 10, or 15 things they have to do. They can't even do one thing well because, while trying to do one thing, their minds remain preoccupied with something else. What can you do about this? Change your approach. Drop everything from your mind but the thing at hand. Concentrate on the immediate task. Center every ounce of your attention on it.

If your mind begins to wander, stop. Stop everything. For example, let's say you're trying to read something and your mind is thinking a hundred different things. Stop. Stop your reading immediately. Tell your mind, "Okay, you want to think about these hundred different things, I'll give you five minutes, then I want your entire attention focused on this article I'm reading." Give the mind five minutes. Listen to all the thoughts. Take each thought one at a time, thoughts about dishes not getting done, about why you're not working at a higher paying job, about guilt over some inadvertent statement you made to a friend last week, about getting the lawn mowed, or about some sexual need you have. Give each thought its due until you've reviewed your entire mental list of distractions. Then get back to your reading.

Practice paying attention. Focus your mind. To do this, try batting away all thoughts that interfere. Visualize yourself using a baseball bat to knock each intruding thought out of your mind.

Do one thing at a time. If you're going to eat, eat. If you're going to talk, talk. If you're going to hammer a nail, hammer a nail. Do nothing else but the thing at hand. You'll get much more done that way and have far better results.

ALL THINGS COME TO THOSE WHO WAIT

This saying comes from the East; in the West, we say, "Patience is a virtue." Both mean the same thing, except the Eastern saying more aptly describes what you need to do.

You need to wait. It's something you must learn.

You might want a lot of things in your life, and you might want many things right now. Indeed, you might get impatient waiting for things to happen. But if you try to force things to happen, you will not succeed. You cannot get what you want by forcing.

Deep inside, you must be ready for changes. It takes time. You must be mature enough in your life to handle certain kinds of benefits, including financial success.

If you learn to wait for what you want, you'll work toward it gradually and change accordingly. Then one day it will happen. It will come to you. The thing you have wanted and waited for will be yours.

So relax. Be patient. And wait.

OLD ENDINGS ARE NEW BEGINNINGS

As one thing ends, something new begins. This is true of everything in the universe, including everything inside of you.

So as you change, drop the old and make way for the new. Remember to leave the past in the past. Open yourself to the new. Don't linger over losses; instead, consider what you're gaining that's new.

As one thing ends, enjoy your adventure. Something new will soon begin. Get ready for it. The moment of discovery awaits.

EVERYTHING CHANGES

Everything changes all the time. Nothing remains the same—even for a moment. Realize this and you can go with it instead of fighting against it.

Whenever we resist change, whenever we refuse to change, we stagnate. Inside we become stuck, brittle, and unhealthy. But the more we go with changes, the more we allow ourselves to change—the more we grow. Experiencing changes, we renew ourselves, we refresh ourselves, and we become wise.

So be flexible in your life. Allow yourself to change. Go with the flow. Meditate on change itself until, through the meditation, you become one with the ever-changing world around you.

DON'T TAKE ANYTHING TOO SERIOUSLY

This so-called universe appears as a juggling,
a picture show. To be happy, look upon it so.
        —Tantric saying

Nothing in this universe has much meaning beyond what the mind sees in it. Actually, the mind attaches too much meaning to things. Relax the mind, and the world changes.

In our lives, we get, at best, only glimpses of reality, fleeting moments of meaning. When allowed to do so, the mind can just as easily find no meaning. At any given moment, one thing might seem true, yet the opposite might also seem true.

When you look at the world on one level, you might see meaning. When you look at the world on another level, you might see no meaning at all. But when you view the world on both levels at the same time, you might well burst out in laughter.

LIVE THIS VERY MOMENT

How do you know what's happening now? Think about it and you lose it. Why? Too many thoughts clutter your vision.

Try this: Drop all thoughts of the future. Drop all thoughts of the past. Say nothing to yourself. Form no sentences, no words. What's left? Receptivity to all that's around you. Oneness—you become one with the world each and every moment.

Here's a simple practice: Choose anything (the grass, the sky, a tree, or anything you like). Meditate on it—become one with it. Allow yourself to merge with it and it to merge with you. Feel it fully. Now notice that your mind is still. If your mind so much as says a word, you lose the moment. If your mind says "green," you lose the grass.

This is what meditation is all about—quieting the mind. The mind chatters on and on, endlessly. If you can drop your mind, you can gain the moment. By opening yourself in this way, each moment feels infinite.

Now consider what it would be like . . .

> To see a World in a Grain of Sand
> And a Heaven in a Wild Flower,
> Hold Infinity in the palm of your hand
> And Eternity in an hour.
>
> —From a poem by
> William Blake

YOU CAN'T HAVE EVERYTHING ALL AT ONCE

People want things—many things. We all desire something more than what we have. Yet desire causes pain.

Why? Because you desire only things you don't have. This means that you feel a lack—that something is missing—and that causes pain.

Desire means that you feel incomplete. You need something more. Ideally, you would like to have everything all at once. It would make you feel complete. Yet you can't have everything all at once. It's impossible. It can never happen. You'll always want something more.

The root of the problem is desire itself. So here's what to do: Drop desire. Stop wanting more and more. Drop it. It's desire that hurts. It's that need for something more that makes you feel incomplete.

You don't need the new sports car, the new love, the hundred thousand dollars, or the new pair of shoes, to make you feel complete. Drop your desires, and you'll feel whole exactly the way you are. One person, one integrity.

HEAR THE TRUTH WITHIN

Open yourself to the inner sanctum. Open yourself to your body. Go inside and listen to what your body tells you and be sensitive to every detail. Don't get stuck in your mind. Remember, the brain is just one of many organs in your body. When you need to think, use this organ. Otherwise, don't think. Just feel. Use your body to feel.

Inside, your body holds incredible wisdom, and it's up to you to discover it. How can you do that? Become quiet with yourself. Become your body. Hear your body from deep within and let it tell you what you need.

YOUR LIFE IS AS LONG
AS YOU WANT IT TO BE

When you quit the drugs, your life opens up to you—totally and completely. No longer does your life seem to be a whirlwind affair, passing you by.

When you quit, it seems like time slows down. You begin living more in every moment. Consequently, your whole life seems to transcend time. You begin to feel as if you're living in eternity.

Life has no boundaries now. You'll live longer in actual number of years, and you'll be in better health. In fact, the more attention you pay to your health, the more years you'll add to your life.

But now, you experience something even more interesting: Each moment of your life feels limitless. Each moment feels vast, greater than the moments you've known before. Now, as the moments grow long, your life grows long. Each new moment is significant and within each moment, your life is as long as you want it to be.

YOU CAN HAVE THIS DAY FOR FREE

Let's face it: On certain days, things go wrong. On some days everything seems to go wrong.

What can you do? One answer: Simply write it off. Things will be better tomorrow or the next day. But today, don't worry. You can have this day for free.

Already you've gained a hundred days a hundred ways. Simply by quitting the drugs, you've added years to your life. Plus, by taking good care of yourself and improving your health, you'll add extra days to your life on a regular basis.

Yes, you will live longer.

So now, whenever you need to, take a free day. Just give yourself the day. Allow the day to go any way it will. Don't even worry if nothing gets done. If you're having a bad day, write it off. If you simply need a break, take it. Either way, just let the day go in utter happiness. You'll have another day to make up for it.

CHAPTER 15

Making Your Life a Success

> *"Would you tell me, please, which way I ought to go from here?"*
>
> *"That depends a good deal on where you want to get to," said the Cat.*
>
> *"I don't much care where—" said Alice.*
>
> *"Then it doesn't matter which way you go," said the Cat.*
>
> *"—so long as I get somewhere," Alice added as an explanation.*
>
> *"Oh, you're sure to do that," said the Cat, "if only you walk long enough."*
>
> —Lewis Carroll, from
> Alice's Adventures in
> Wonderland

Here's your big payoff. You have made major changes. You have fought a long, hard battle. You might even have gone through great difficulties to get here. But you have won.

Now you're starting to control your own life. Indeed, your life has become more manageable than ever. And because of this, you can raise your sights. Now you can pick your own goals and achieve them. If you apply the right amount of effort, you can achieve almost any goal you choose.

WHAT ARE YOUR IMPORTANT GOALS?

The more you reclaim your life from drugs (and other addictions), the more you can achieve. By dropping your addictions, you become stronger and more in control of your life. Success is then more likely.

It doesn't happen all at once. It happens in steps. By quitting the drugs, you take a giant step toward personal growth and improvement. By quitting other addictions (alcohol, nicotine, caffeine, sugar, or over-eating), you gain even more power. As you clear away these obstacles, your life transforms miraculously, and success becomes inevitable.

What do you choose to do? Think about it. It's good to know what you want, what you're aiming for. How can you hit a target if you can't see it? In Worksheet #15, you'll list some goals that are important to you. Then, at the end of this chapter, you'll learn specific ways to achieve these goals.

Worksheet #15

Personal Life Goals

Instructions. Write your personal goals. Be realistic. For each type of goal, write what you would like to accomplish in one year, in five years, in your lifetime. Take your time. If you're not sure of your goals in a specific area, come back to it later. Describe your goals as you see them today. But remember, your goals will probably change over time, so review this chart regularly and revise it as necessary.

Goals	1-Year Goal	5-Year Goal	Lifetime Goal
Physical			
•Appearance	_____	_____	_____
•Health	_____	_____	_____
Mental			
•Clarity	_____	_____	_____
•Creativity	_____	_____	_____
•Attitude	_____	_____	_____
Emotional			
•Calmness	_____	_____	_____
•Happiness	_____	_____	_____
•Self-confidence	_____	_____	_____
Spiritual			
•Renewed faith	_____	_____	_____
•Inner peace	_____	_____	_____
Social			
•Strangers	_____	_____	_____
•Acquaintances	_____	_____	_____
•Friends	_____	_____	_____
Family			
•Spouse	_____	_____	_____
•Children	_____	_____	_____
•Mother	_____	_____	_____
•Father	_____	_____	_____
•Brother(s)	_____	_____	_____
•Sister(s)	_____	_____	_____
Career			
•Job	_____	_____	_____
•Business venture	_____	_____	_____
Financial	_____	_____	_____
Education	_____	_____	_____

Sports/fitness	_____	_____	_____
Diet	_____	_____	_____
Hobbies	_____	_____	_____
Community service	_____	_____	_____
Other	_____	_____	_____

GETTING WHAT YOU WANT AND GETTING GOOD RESULTS WITHOUT DRUGS

At this moment, you're in a good position. By quitting the drugs, you've proven yourself capable of achieving a goal. This means that you've dealt with, and overcome, obstacles along the way. But that's not all. Now that you've quit using drugs, you've gotten rid of a major obstacle that has prevented you from achieving important life goals.

In Worksheet #15, you listed personal life goals that are important to you. That's the beginning because once you know your goals, you can begin doing what's necessary to achieve them. So, what's necessary?

Zig Ziglar, a renowned teacher of goal achievement, travels the country giving dynamic talks on goal achievement and how to be a winner. (Some of Zig's talks have been videotaped and are available from Nightingale-Conant Corporation at 800-525-9000. I recommend that you order the one titled "GOALS.") Zig presents seven steps to achieving goals:

1. Identify your goal.
2. Set a deadline.
3. List obstacles you must overcome.

4. Identify people who can help and get them to help you.

5. List the skills you need to accomplish your goal. Obtain these skills.

6. Develop a plan and write it down.

7. List the benefits of achieving your goal.

Now write your seven steps for each goal that you listed in Worksheet #15. Then follow the steps. Start following your plan for each of your goals. By working toward your goals in this manner, you will be successful.

CHAPTER 16

Freedom

I only ask to be free. The butterflies are free.
—*Charles Dickens*

A h, freedom: what we won't do to get it—but how easy it is to lose.

Drugs take your freedom away. Chained to the addiction, you can hardly go anywhere without being concerned about your drug supply. Some heavy users can't even go for a ride to a nearby store without first catching a buzz.

Deep in the addiction, your whole life becomes tied to the drugs. You can't even get up in the morning or wake up in the middle of the night without needing to use. In one case, you need the drugs to wake you up; in the other case, you need them to put you back to sleep.

At this stage of addiction, the drugs control you. You're stuck. It's like half of your life is gone, and whole parts of you are no longer available to you. It's like half of you is already dead and buried.

That's why everybody addicted to drugs, deep down inside, wants to quit. The reasons are clear. Quitting drugs will set you free. Quitting drugs will make you whole again. Quitting drugs will give you new breath, new life, and new hope for happiness. What more could you ask for?

FEELING FREE

Life changes when you quit using drugs. Have you noticed? You've become free, perhaps freer than you've ever known. But along with freedom comes responsibility.

With drugs, you were often irresponsible. Many basic responsibilities—keeping a job, meeting the needs of your family, meeting your own needs, treating other people with respect, and so on—were just too much for you. What's worse, you even used drugs as an excuse: "I couldn't help it, I was just a little too high."

Now you have no excuses. Now you're out in the open, on your own. How do you handle the responsibility?

Easy. Simply get right into it.

You have just reclaimed a big part of your life. Now it's time to live and watch how things change. When you become so completely involved in every aspect of your life, you begin enjoying it fully. Life's responsibilities soon become life's pleasures.

You begin to like your work—even if it takes changing your job—and you begin to succeed at it. You feel good about meeting the needs of your family, especially their emotional needs. You begin to feel good about yourself as you regain your physical and emotional health. And you begin to enjoy other people. You start showing respect for other people, and—the big reward—they start respecting you.

So how do you deal with open spaces? Step right in. Do what's needed. Once in a while, do something silly just for fun. Stay with your program, but above all enjoy yourself.

STEERING CLEAR OF TROUBLE

To free oneself is nothing; it is being free that is hard.

—Andre Gide

If you stay goal-directed and keep working toward your goals, you'll keep your freedom. Sure, you can take a day off once in a while, but nearly every day you need to work toward your goals.

Does this sound like a grind? Like there's no fun involved? Maybe it sounds hard, but remember: When you achieve your goals, you gain many benefits. For example, if one of your goals is to lose weight, you'll begin hearing compliments from other people, you'll begin feeling better inside, you'll enjoy greater health, and you'll live longer. Losing weight might be work, it might even be hard work, but the benefits are worth it.

So keep your perspective on things—and keep your course.

Practice #9

Three Ways to Keep Your Freedom

Do these three things to help maintain your freedom:

- Keep rewarding yourself: Give yourself gifts, rewards, and prizes on a regular basis (at least one every two weeks). To find something new or to recall your favorite rewards, go over Checklist #6 in Chapter 13.

- Review your benefits again and again: Over the course of your life, you continually gain new and different benefits by not using drugs. Knowing these benefits helps you to stay off the drugs. So review your list of benefits (Worksheet #14 in Chapter 13) often, maybe every two months, and add to it as necessary.

• Check your life goals regularly: Review your progress toward these goals. As you achieve them, write down the benefits you experience. Have your goals changed? If so, revise Worksheet #15 in Chapter 15. Review your goals and your progress toward your goals on a regular basis, maybe twice a month.

A NEW YOU

Who are you now? Without drugs changing your body chemistry, don't you feel like a different person? Aren't you more mature, more capable, more kind, more loving?

Yes, you are.

Of course, you'll have some days when you feel bad. But keep in mind the fact that they will pass. Overall, you keep gaining ground, changing inside, and discovering something new about yourself.

In fact, when you quit the drugs, you assume a new identity. You start becoming someone new. Indeed, the transformation is so complete that you actually become a different person.

So go with this. Get yourself up to it. Enjoy the changes and enjoy the new you.

For fun, you might even want to change your name. It might be something as simple as asking to be called Michael instead of Mike or Susan instead of Susie. Tell your family and friends. You might also want to get rid of drug-related nicknames. For example, you might prefer Martin to Sharp-Shooter, Jenna to Joy-Popper, Rose to Roadie, Sam to Electroglide, or Barb to Biscuit. Or you might want to choose a brand-new name—maybe even something personally important or symbolic to you.

Meanwhile, you may or may not want to call yourself an "addict." If you decide not to refer to yourself as an addict, that's fine. For practical purposes, you're not an addict when you're not using. On the other hand you may prefer to call yourself an addict or a "recovering addict" because it gives you a constant reminder that you cannot use drugs. That's fine, too, as it serves a useful purpose.

Whatever your choice, be sure to acknowledge the new you. Open yourself to a changing pattern. Drop the old addicted part of you. Let the new you shine through.

In the old self, you were constrained. In the new self, you're open to all the world. In the old self, drugs kept you locked in a box. In the new self, someone has opened the box—and now you're free.

Indeed, you've opened the box yourself. You've quit using drugs on your own, and you deserve a great deal of praise. You've become a success to yourself and to many other people around you.

Good work.

Keep it up.

Afterword

Congratulations.

You've shown the courage to change. There were probably times when it wasn't easy, but you've worked hard, and you've become a success. You deserve a great amount of credit.

Now you can begin enjoying your life more fully. You've grown. You've opened the door to many additional opportunities, and you have more choices than ever. You've gained your freedom.

I encourage you to continue your success. I feel certain that you can—and I feel confident that you will.

Now, if you have a moment, I would like to hear from you. Over the years, I've conducted hundreds of interviews with folks who had problems with drugs and alcohol. I've developed what I think is the best program to meet everyone's needs. But tell me, how well did the program work for you? What methods worked best? What ideas do you have to help me improve this book?

On the other hand, if you want help with a specific problem, or if you want me to answer any questions you might have, I'm available. I'll send you a response as soon as possible.

Feel free to write to me:

Jerry Dorsman
c/o New Dawn
P.O. Box 71
Elk Mills, MD 21920

Bibliography and Recommended Reading

AA World Services. *Alcoholics Anonymous*. New York: AA World Services, Inc., 1955.

⸺⸺⸺⸺. *Comments on AA's Triennial Surveys.* New York: AA World Services, Inc., 1990.

Airola, Paavo, N.D., Ph.D. *Hypoglycemia: A Better Approach*. Phoenix, AZ: Health Plus Publishers, 1977.

Alberti, Robert, Ph.D., and Emmons, Michael, Ph.D. *Your Perfect Right: A Guide to Assertive Living*. San Luis Obispo, CA: Impact Publishers, 1990.

American Lung Association. *Freedom from Smoking in 20 Days*. Washington, D.C.: American Lung Association, 1980.

Anderson, Bob. *Stretching*. Bolinas, CA: Shelter Publications, 1980.

Annand, Margo. *The Art of Sexual Ecstasy*. Los Angeles: Jeremy P. Tarcher, 1989.

Beasley, Joseph, M.D., and Knightly, Susan. *Food for Recovery: The Complete Nutritional Companion for Recovering from Alcoholism, Drug Abuse, and Eating Disorders*. New York: Crown Publishers, 1994.

Buscaglia, Leo. *Love*. New York: Ballantine Books, 1972.

Chang, Jolan. *The Tao of Love and Sex*. London: Wildwood House, 1977.

Christopher, James. *Unhooked: Staying Sober and Drug-Free*. Buffalo, NY: Prometheus Books, 1989.

_____. *SOS Sobriety: The Proven Alternative to 12-Step Programs.* Buffalo, NY: Prometheus Books, 1992.

Colbin, Annemarie. *Food and Healing.* New York: Ballantine Books, 1986.

Cousens, Gabriel, M.D. "Living Food." *New Frontier Magazine.* September 1989.

Devereaux, Paul. *The Long Trip: A Prehistory of Psychedelia.* New York: Arkana/Penguin, 1997.

Douglas, Nik, and Slinger, Penny. *Sexual Secrets.* New York: Destiny Books, 1979.

Drug Enforcement Administration of the U.S. Department of Justice. *Drugs of Abuse* (1997 ed.). Arlington, VA: Drug Enforcement Administration, 1997.

Dufty, William. *Sugar Blues.* New York: Warner Books, 1975.

Esko, Edward, and Esko, Wendy. *Macrobiotic Cooking for Everyone.* Tokyo: Japan Publications, Inc., 1980.

Fanning, Patrick, and O'Neill, John T., L.C.D.C. *The Addiction Workbook: A Step-by-Step Guide to Quitting Alcohol and Drugs.* Oakland, CA: New Harbinger, 1996.

Fields, Rick; Taylor, Peggy; Weyler, Rex; and Ingrasci, Rick. *Chop Wood, Carry Water: A Guide to Finding Spiritual Fulfillment in Everyday Life.* Los Angeles: Jeremy P. Tarcher, 1984.

Finnegan, John, and Gray, Daphne. *Recovery from Addiction.* Berkeley, CA: Celestial Arts, 1990.

Fischer-Rizzi, Susanne. *Medicine of the Earth.* Portland, OR: Rudra Press, 1996.

Folan, Lilias M. *Lilias, Yoga and You.* New York: Bantam Books, 1972.

Foundation for Inner Peace. *A Course in Miracles.* Tiburon, CA: Foundation for Inner Peace, 1975.

Gurion, J. "Remaking Our Lives." *American Health.* March 1990.

Health Education Center of the Maryland Department of Health and Mental Hygiene. *Getting Fit Your Way: A Self-Paced Fitness Guide.* Washington, DC: U.S. Government Printing Office, 1983.

Hoskins, Ray. *Rational Madness: The Paradox of Addiction.* Blue Ridge Summit, PA: Tab Books, 1989.

Iceberg Slim. *Pimp: The Story of My Life.* Los Angeles: Hollaway House, 1967.

Irwin, Samuel, Ph.D. *Drugs of Abuse* (booklet). Phoenix, AZ: Do It Now Foundation, 1989.

Jamplonsky, Gerald. *Love is Letting Go of Fear.* New York: Bantam Books, 1981.

Johnson, Vernon E. *I'll Quit Tomorrow.* New York: Harper and Row, 1973.

Ketcham, Katherine, and Mueller, L. Ann, M.D. *Eating Right to Live Sober.* New York: New American Library, 1983.

Kirkpatrick, Jean, Ph.D. *Goodbye Hangovers, Hello Life: Self-Help for Women.* Quakertown, PA: Women for Sobriety, 1996.

_____. *Turnabout: New Help for the Woman Alcoholic.* New York: Bantam Books, 1990.

Kotzsch, Ron. "Are Your Compulsions Out of Control?" *EastWest Journal.* June 1983.

Kuhn, Cynthia; Swartzwelder, Scott; and Wilson, Wilkie. *Buzzed: The Straight Facts About the Most Used and Abused Drugs from Alcohol to Ecstacy.* New York: Norton, 1998.

L'Esperance, Carrie. *The Ancient Cookfire: How to Rejuvenate the Body and Spirit Through Seasonal Foods and Fasting.* Santa Fe, NM: Bear and Co., 1998.

Levant, Glenn. *Keeping Kids Drug Free: D.A.R.E. Official Parents Guide.* San Diego: Laurel Glen, 1998.

Leviton, Richard. "Staying Drugfree Naturally." *EastWest Journal.* March 1988.

Lewis, Judith A. *Addictions: Concepts and Strategies for Treatment.* Gaithersburg, MD: Aspen Publishers, 1994.

Lingeman, Richard R. *Drugs from A to Z: A Dictionary.* New York: McGraw-Hill, 1969.

McLanahan, Amrita Sandra, M.D. "Health, Yoga and Anatomy" (videotape). Buckingham, VA: Integral Yoga Distribution, Satchidananda Ashram.

Milhorn, H. Thomas, Jr., M.D., Ph.D. *Drug and Alcohol Abuse: The Authoritative Guide for Parents, Teachers, and Counselors.* New York: Plenum, 1994.

Miller, William R. (ed.). *The Addictive Behaviors: Treatment of Alcoholism, Drug Abuse, Smoking and Obesity.* New York: Pergamon Press, 1980.

Miller, William R., et al. "What Works: A Methodological Analysis of the Alcohol Treatment Outcome Literature." In *Handbook of Alcoholism Treatment Approaches* (Reid K. Hester and William R. Miller, eds.). Needham Heights, MA: Allyn & Bacon, 1995.

Mindell, Earl. *Earl Mindell's Vitamin Bible.* New York: Rawson, Wade Publishers, 1979.

Mooney, Al J., M.D.; Eisenberg, Arlene; and Eisenberg, Howard. *The Recovery Book.* New York: Workman, 1992.

Mueller, L. Ann, M.D., and Ketcham, Katherine. *Recovering: How to Get and Stay Sober.* New York: Bantam Books, 1987.

Mumey, Jack, and Hatcher, Anne S., Ed.D., R.D. *Good Food for a Sober Life.* Chicago: Contemporary Books, 1987.

Muramoto, Naboru, with Abehsera, Michel. *Healing Ourselves.* New York: Avon, 1973.

Narcotics Anonymous (NA). *Am I an Addict?; Who, What, How, and Why; Welcome to Narcotics Anonymous; Some Thoughts Regarding Our Relationship to Alcoholics Anonymous; and Facts About Narcotics Anonymous: A Society of Recovering Drug Addicts.* Van Nuys, CA: Narcotics Anonymous World Service Office.

National Institute of Drug Abuse. *Assessing Neurotoxicity of Drugs of Abuse.* Bethesda, MD: National Institutes of Health, 1993.

_____. "Drug Abuse and the Brain" (videotape). Bethesda, MD: National Institutes of Health.

_____. *Drugs and the Brain* (booklet). Bethesda, MD: National Institutes of Health.

_____. *Pharmacokinetics, Metabolism, and Pharmaceutics of Drugs of Abuse.* Bethesda, MD: National Institutes of Health, 1997.

Null, Gary, and Null, Steven. *How to Get Rid of the Poisons in Your Body.* New York: Arco, 1977.

O'Connell, David F., and Alexander, Charles N. (eds.). *Self Recovery: Treating Addictions Using Transcendental*

Meditation and Maharishi Ayur-Veda. New York: Haworth Press, 1994.

Orford, Jim. *Excessive Appetites: A Psychological View of Addiction.* New York: Wiley, 1985.

Ott, John. *Health and Light.* New York: Pocket Books, 1976.

Patterson, Meg, M.B.E., M.B.Ch.B., F.R.C.S.E. *Hooked? Net: the New Approach to Drug Cure.* London: Faber and Faber, 1986.

Peele, Stanton, Ph.D., and Brodsky, Archie, with Arnold, Mary. *The Truth About Addiction and Recovery: The Life Process Program for Outgrowing Destructive Habits.* New York: Simon & Schuster, 1991.

Phelps, Janice K., M.D., and Nourse, Alan E., M.D. *The Hidden Addiction: And How to Get Free.* Boston: Little, Brown, 1986.

Porth, Carol. *Pathophysiology, Concepts of Altered Health States.* Philadelphia: Lippincott, 1982.

Pritikin, Nathan, with McGrady, Patric, Jr. *The Pritikin Program for Diet and Exercise.* New York: Grosset & Dunlap, 1973.

Prochaska, James, Ph.D.; Norcross, John, Ph.D.; and DiClemente, Carlo, Ph.D. *Changing for Good: The Revolutionary Program That Explains the Six Stages of Change and Teaches You How to Free Yourself from Bad Habits.* New York: Morrow, 1994.

Rajneesh, Bhagwan Shree. *The Book of Secrets* (5 volumes). New York: Harper and Row, 1974.

Ray, Sondra. *Loving Relationships.* Berkeley, CA: Celestial Arts, 1980.

Robertson, Dr. Joel. *Help Yourself: A Revolutionary Alternative Recovery Program.* Nashville, TN: Thomas Nelson Publishers, 1992.

Robinson, Corrine, and Lawler, Marilyn. *Normal and Therapeutic Nutrition* (16th ed.). New York: Macmillan, 1982.

Rudgley, Richard. *Essential Substances: A Cultural History of Intoxicants in Society.* New York: Kodansha International, 1993.

Saifer, Phyllis, M.D., M.P.H., and Zellerbach, Merla. *Detox.* New York: Ballantine Books, 1984.

Salk, Lee, Ph.D. *Familyhood*. New York: Simon & Schuster, 1992.

Salwak, Dale (ed.). *The Wonders of Solitude*. Novato, CA: New World Library, 1998.

Schaler, Jeffrey A., Ph.D. *Drugs: Should We Legalize, Decriminalize or Deregulate?* Amhurst, NY: Prometheus, 1998.

Seymour, Richard, and Smith, David, M.D. *Drugfree: A Unique, Positive Approach to Staying Off Alcohol and Other Drugs*. New York: Facts on File, 1987.

Siegel, Bernie. *Love, Medicine and Miracles*. New York: Harper and Row, 1986.

Smith, Manuel J. *When I Say No, I Feel Guilty*. New York: Bantam Books, 1975.

Substance Abuse and Mental Health Services Administration of the U.S. Department of Health and Human Services. *Detoxification from Alcohol and Other Drugs*. Rockville, MD: SAMHSA, 1995.

_____.*50 Strategies for Substance Abuse Treatment*. Rockville, MD: SAMHSA, 1997.

_____. *National Household Survey on Drug Abuse: Population Estimates 1996*. Rockville, MD: SAMHSA, 1997.

_____. *The Prevalence and Correlates of Treatment for Drug Problems*. Rockville, MD: SAMHSA, 1997.

_____. *Trends in the Incidence of Drug Use in the United States, 1919–1992*. Rockville, MD: SAMHSA, 1996.

Tierra, Michael, G.A., N.D. *The Way of Herbs*. New York: Washington Square Press, 1980.

Tracy, Lisa. *The Gradual Vegetarian*. New York: Dell, 1985.

Trimpey, Jack. *Rational Recovery: The New Cure for Substance Addiction*. New York: Pocket Books, 1996.

Tortera, Gerald; Funke, Berdell; and Case, Christine. *Microbiology: An Introduction*. Menlo Park, CA: Benjamin/Cummings Publishing, 1982.

Tyler, Andrew. *Street Drugs: The Facts Explained, the Myths Exploded* (rev. ed.). London: Hodder and Stroughton, 1995.

Walters, Glenn D. *Substance Abuse and the New Road to Recovery*. Bristol, PA: Taylor & Francis, 1996.

Weil, A., and Rosen, W. *From Chocolate to Morphine: Everything You Need to Know About Mind-Altering Substances*. New York: Houghton Mifflin, 1993.

Williams, Dr. Roger J. *The Prevention of Alcoholism Through Nutrition*. New York: Bantam Books, 1981.

Worwood, Susan. *Essential Aromatherapy*. San Raphael, CA: New World Library, 1995.

Index

About the Author

Jerry Dorsman, B.A.C., developed his highly successful recovery program over a 14-year period. During this time, he researched and tested hundreds of techniques that can help individuals break their addictions to alcohol and drugs. This research culminated in 1991 with the publication of his first book, *How to Quit Drinking Without AA*.

His original goal was to help himself. In his personal life, he had struggled with addictions to alcohol and numerous drugs. By 1981, he broke the last of these addictions, the one to alcohol.

In its first edition, *How to Quit Drinking Without AA* quickly became a top-selling recovery title. An updated and revised edition was published by Prima Publishing in 1994. By 1998, this self-help guide had sold more than 65,000 copies. Also, two foreign-language editions—in Spanish and in Russian—have been released for distribution in 1993 and 1997, respectively.

His second book, *You Can Achieve Peace of Mind* (Prima, 1994), was coauthored with stress management therapist Bob Davis. This book presents over 140 methods that individuals can use to attain a calm inner state.

As an expert on addiction and addiction treatment, Jerry has appeared on more than 125 radio shows all over the United States and Canada and on three local television shows. In addition, articles about his addiction treatment program, including book reviews, have appeared in *USA Today*, *The Chicago Tribune*, *The Philadelphia Inquirer*, *Your Health* magazine (cover story), *Natural Health* magazine, *Better World* magazine, and almost every magazine, newsletter, and newsmagazine in the field of addiction and recovery. Jerry has written articles on recovery that have appeared in *The Counselor, Behavioral Health Management, Professional Counselor, Addiction & Recovery, Journal of Rational Recovery, The Northeast Recovery Networker,* and *Journey.*

Jerry is certified as an addictions counselor and holds two academic degrees. He has worked as a drug and alcohol counselor, as the director of a drug and alcohol counseling center in Pennsylvania, as a mental health counselor, and as the director of many mental health programs in Maryland. Currently, he works for Upper Bay Counseling and Support Services in Cecil County, Maryland, where, aside from administrative responsibilities, he provides therapy for mental health clients who have problems with drug and alcohol addictions.